Sixth Edition

Notter's Essentials of Nursing Research

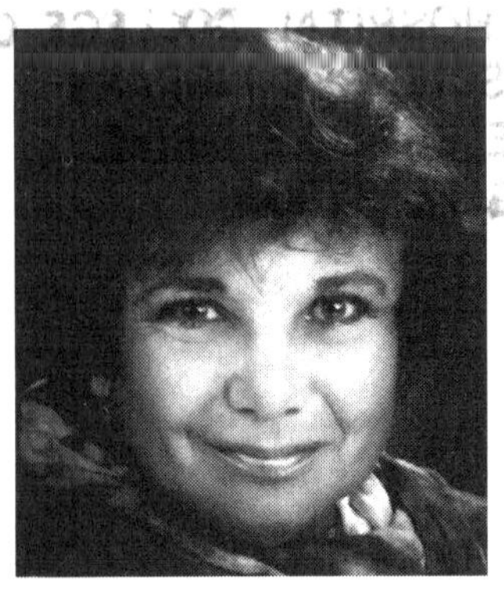

Jacqueline Rose Hott, RN, CS, PhD, FAAN, is Dean and Professor Emerita of Adelphi University School of Nursing and was Co-Director of the Project for Research in Nursing, Adelphi University, 1977 to 1982; Executive Director, Mid-Atlantic Regional Nursing Association (MARNA), 1982 to 1985; and Chair, American Nurses Association (ANA) Council of Nurse Researchers, 1985 to 1987. She was elected to the American Academy of Nursing in 1978 and nominated for the Excellence in Research Award, National Founders Award of Sigma Theta Tau in 1983. Dr. Hott was named a "Women with Clout" by *The Women's Record* in January 1986 and received the First Mentor Award from Sigma Theta Tau, Alpha Omega Chapter, and the Distinguished Alumni Award from the New York University Division of Nursing Alumni in 1987; she was most recently honored by Soroptimist International of Nassau County with the "Women Helping Women" Award. She served as a member of the New York State Nurses Association Council on Nursing Research, 1990 to 1994. She serves as a distinguished lecturer for Sigma Theta Tau International. She also serves on the Advisory Board for the Adelphi University School of Nursing and for the Center for Nursing Research and Scholarly Practice at Molloy College. Dr. Hott is certified by the ANA as a clinical specialist in adult psychiatric mental health nursing and is certified in sex therapy by the American Association of Sex Educators, Counselors, and Therapists (AASECT). She holds postdoctoral certification in psychoanalysis and psychotherapy from Adelphi University Derner Institute and has served as president of the Northeast Psychological Associates. She is a sex therapist on the staff of New York University Behavioral Therapy Program.

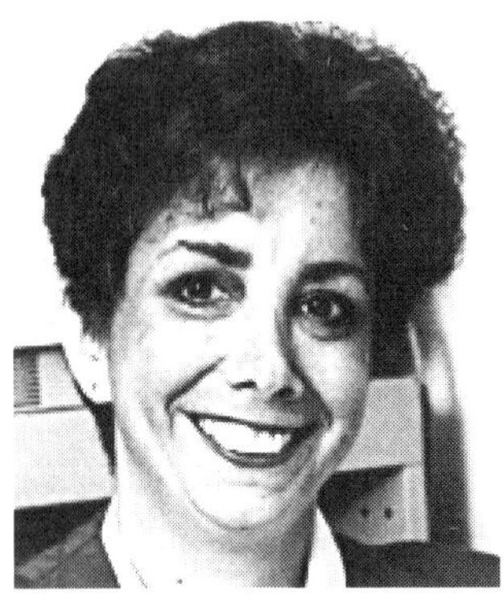

Wendy C. Budin, PhD, RN,C, is Assistant Professor of Nursing and Program Director of the Lamaze International Childbirth Educator Certification Program at Seton Hall University. She received one of the first NJ Breast Cancer Visiting Research Scholar Fellowships, awarded by the NJ State Commission on Cancer Research, 1996, to work with Dr. Carol Noll Hoskins, Professor of Nursing, New York University (NYU), on research dealing with adjustment to breast cancer. Dr. Budin's research "Psychosocial Adjustment to Breast Cancer in Unmarried Women" was funded by a grant from the American Nurses Foundation, and she was named the 1994 ANF Barbara A. Given Scholar. For this research, she also received the 1997 Sigma Theta Tau International Regional Research Dissertation Award. Other awards include the Distinguished Alumnus Award, Nursing Alumni Council, Seton Hall University, 1998; the NYU Arch Award, 1996 and Division of Nursing, Rudin Award, 1995; Excellence in Research Award, Sigma Theta Tau, Gamma Nu Chapter, 1991; and Faculty Role Model from the graduating class of Seton Hall College of Nursing, 1996, 1997. Dr. Budin is certified as a perinatal nurse by The American Nurses Credentialing Center (ANCC). Dr. Budin was appointed to the Joint Nursing/Psychosocial Advisory Group to the NJ State Commission on Cancer Research, the Education/Research Committee and Certification Council of Lamaze International and is a consultant for Regents College, The University of the State of New York, in the content area of Research in Nursing.

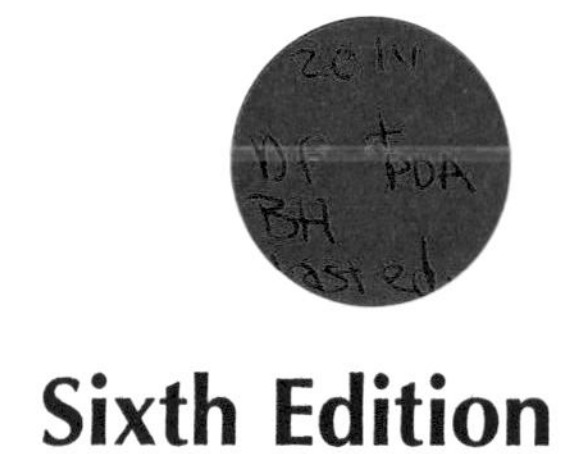

Sixth Edition

Notter's Essentials of Nursing Research

Jacqueline Rose Hott, RN, CS, PhD, FAAN
Wendy C. Budin, PhD, RN, C

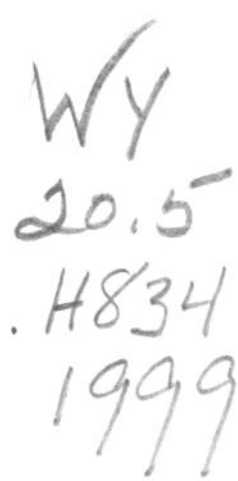

 Springer Publishing Company

Springer Publishing Company, Inc.
536 Broadway
New York, NY 10012-3955

Cover design by Janet Joachim
Acquisitions Editor: Sheri W. Sussman
Production Editor: Pamela Lankas

99 00 01 02 03 / 5 4 3 2 1

Library of Congress Cataloging-in-Publication-Data

Hott, Jacqueline Rose.
Notter's essentials of nursing research / by Jacqueline Rose Hott and Wendy C. Budin. — 6th ed.
p. cm.
Rev. ed. of: Essentials of nursing research / Lucille E. Notter, Jacqueline Rose Hott. 5th ed.c1994.
Includes bibliographical references and index.
ISBN 0-8261-1599-3
1. Nursing—Research. I. Budin, Wendy C. II. Notter, Lucille E. (Lucille Elizabeth), 1907–1993. Essentials of nursing research. III. Title
[DNLM: 1. Nursing Research. WY 20.5H834n 1999]
RT81.5.N67 1999
610.73'07'2—dc21
DNLM/DLC
for Library of Congress 98-39259
CIP

Printed in the United States of America

Contents

III Evaluation of Research

Foreword

This new edition of *Notter's Essentials of Nursing Research* provides a contemporary explanation of the basic knowledge and skills that form the foundation of nursing research of clinical practice. The authors, Hott and Budin, expand the original work with examples of nursing research that enrich the text and, in particular, clarify the essential content. This book thus serves as an excellent introductory text for students in their first professional degree program and for beginning graduate students in nursing.

Further, this publication is timely in that nursing research has come of age. Research courses are part of the curricula of all educational programs. Clinical nurse researchers are employed by many health care agencies and systems; the nursing research budget within the National Institutes of Health National Institute of Nursing Research has grown steadily, and evidence-based practice is the expectation within nursing and health care. All professional nurses are now expected to be familiar not only with the language of research, but also with the underlying rationale for integration of research findings into professional practice. This book provides the important introductory information.

There are many attractive features of this new edition that will convince the student to continue to use the book throughout his or her career. For example, the authors include a glossary of research terms and useful references for obtaining funds for research, from small pilot funds to sources of major support. Other major components of this text that will be of great interest to both novice researchers and teachers of beginning researchers are the references on presenting and publishing research, including how to write a research abstract. Basic facts about key nursing research journals also are presented. And for the newly initiated into the communication age of the Internet, the authors provide a comprehensive list of Web sites for nursing-research activities. All of these special touches, combined with the basics of nursing research, help to make this book a complete resource for the beginner.

Dr. Lucille Notter, the original author of this research text for nurses, would be proud of this newest edition. The straightforward writing style and excellent examples of today's leading nursing research make this an important work for the discipline. But, most especially, it is an important resource for nurses everywhere who are just being introduced to the scientific values that serve as the foundation for professional practice.

JOYCE J. FITZPATRICK, Editor
Annual Review of Nursing Research Series
Encylclopedia of Nursing Research

Preface

Nurses are assuming increasingly demanding professional responsibilities in the health care system, and with this responsibility comes the expectation that they will take a more active role in improving the delivery of health care. What nursing techniques work best for patients? What new procedures are most effective? Research can help us find scientific answers to these questions and other problems in nursing. This book is intended as an introduction to nursing research.

Every nurse has a part to play in nursing research, whether it be as a participant in the research itself, as a user of the products of research, or as someone who identifies problem areas needing research. The research nurse and the practitioner have a common goal: to provide the best nursing care possible. Ideally, they join forces to work toward that goal. Therefore, all professional nurses should be familiar with at least the essentials of nursing research.

Clinical studies (called applied research) aimed at improved practice and better patient care and basic research aimed at expanding the frontiers of knowledge are needed for the development and testing of nursing theories. Although an increasing number of specially qualified nurses are engaged in both clinical and basic research, it is important for all nurses to be aware of this need and to participate to the extent that they can. Many nurses in clinical practice are becoming interested in doing their own research. In addition to participating in research by keeping abreast of new studies, identifying clinical problems for future research, and cooperating and collaborating with research projects initiated in their institutions, these nurses are seeking help in developing the skills required to carry out their own simple but carefully designed studies in the clinical setting. Some institutions now employ research consultants whose function is to stimulate and guide nurses in the conduct of such studies. These small, less sophisticated studies, which have been called "research with a small r" (Ramshorn, 1972), will be done by many nurses with only elementary skills in research—practitioners and clinicians whose intellectual curiosity and spirit of inquiry lead them to observe problems at first hand, define them, and begin to study them. The results of their efforts may inspire them and others to do more comprehensive, sophisticated studies of the additional problems or questions they bring to light.

A major problem that has plagued nursing research arises when many nurses report on clinical studies involving relatively small samples and end their reports by recommending that "further study of the problem" is done, and the impetus achieved is lost. Fortunately, some nurses do continue to study the problem in which they are interested. They study it over time under similar and different conditions and in similar or different settings. These researchers are most likely to make a contribution to scientific knowledge in nursing (Harrer, 1987).*

Eventually, the findings of research must be applied in practice if they are to effect improvement in patient care. This goal can be achieved only if practicing nurses are aware of research projects being carried out and can read and evaluate the findings in terms of their implications for nursing care. Research-oriented nurses should be able to make the most effective use of the findings of research in their daily practice.

This book is an attempt to present the complex process of scientific research simply and concisely to undergraduate students of nursing and to graduate nurses who have had little prior preparation in research methods. This edition, like the past five editions, presents the basics of how to use, perform, and evaluate research in a way useful to those beginning their acquaintance with nursing research. A number of additions have been made in the sixth edition to update and expand the content and to include examples of studies reported in the more recent literature. Attention to qualitative research has been enhanced, and a new chapter devoted to the use of computers in nursing research has been added. We hope this research primer will help nurses begin an involvement with research, which in turn is an involvement with the advancement of the profession.

JACQUELINE ROSE HOTT
WENDY C. BUDIN

REFERENCES

Harrer, K. B. (1987). Reading research for practice. *Maternal Child Nursing, 12,* 226.

Ramshorn, M. (1972). Small *r* in nursing research: An exploratory study of patient experiences in isolation. *Journal of New York State Nurses Association, 3,* 24–29.

---

* See Harrer (1987).

Acknowledgments

As in the two prior editions, I wish to express deep appreciation to the late Dr. Lucille Notter for the opportunity to revise her classic book. Sadly, she was ill and hospitalized during that time and died March 4, 1993, as the fifth edition was being copy edited. I have tried to maintain the very special flair of her personality throughout the subsequent work. It is a truism that as teachers we are taught by our students, and I have been particularly fortunate having Dr. Wendy C. Budin, my former student at Adelphi University School of Nursing, join me as a coauthor for this edition. She brings a freshness and scholarly approach plus clinical expertise to this text, especially in her use of computer technology, which has been invaluable. I welcome her with joy as a coauthor. Further, I want to thank former research assistants Dr. Susan Mayer and Dr. Joyce Fine for their work on the forth and fifth editions, respectively, which laid the groundwork for the current book. Dr. Mayer along with Dr. Susan Buchholtz also contributed additions to the sections on historical research in this edition. Other contributors to whom we express gratitude are Dr. Rose Schecter for clinical applications and Dr. Holly Shaw and Dr. Patricia Munhall for their contributions on qualitative research. Thanks to the people at Springer Publishing, Sheri Sussman, Ruth Chasek, Louise Farkas, and Ursula Springer for their persistence and confidence. To Tim and Sandy, Larry and Diane, Sue and Michael, and Rachel and Steve, and my 10 grandchildren, and my significant others for your patience, understanding, caring, and love in difficult times. . . . I couldn't have done it without you.

JACQUELINE ROSE HOTT

I wish to express a special note of gratitude to Dr. Jacqueline Rose Hott, my long-time mentor and inspiration, for the unique opportunity to work with her on the revisions of this classic book. She has played a most significant role in my professional and personal life, and I thank her from the bottom of my heart for all she has done. I thank each and every one of my good friends and colleagues at Seton Hall University and New York University for their encouragement and support. A special note of thanks to all my students who asked challenging questions and provided enthusiastic feedback and suggestions on how to make learning research more interesting. No words can express my appreciation to my husband Arnie and daughters, Barri, Sarah, and Jill. I realize that at times my preoccupation with my work has not been easy for them. Their inexhaustible patience, understanding, and pride in my accomplishments will always be cherished.

WENDY C. BUDIN

PART I

Introduction to Research

1

Evolution of the Research Movement in Nursing

From the beginning of time, questions have been raised about our human experiences and activities. Answers have been sought to help us understand and deal with the problems that humans encounter. As nurses, we too have become interested in research, because we want to find answers to scientific questions that trouble us. All kinds of nurses, as well as the general public, have raised questions about our education and our practice. How do we know what we know? Why do we do what we do?

Historically, several main approaches have been used to explain phenomena: magic, authority, tradition, logical reasoning, and scientific method. Over the years, nurses have used all these approaches to explain activities or solve problems.

Primitive humans relied on magic or the influence of some supernatural power for an explanation of facts that they could not understand. Later, wise men or authorities were consulted to provide the answers that were needed. Because of their experience or their ability to think through problems and formulate answers, they were counted on to give valid opinions. Authorities, or experts, continue to be used. This is legitimate practice in many instances, at times because answers are needed immediately and there is no time for research and at times because the resources or tools needed to do the required research are not available. It must be remembered, however, that authorities may not always give the best answers, and on occasion, they may give incomplete or even incorrect answers.

The use of tradition is another approach to solving problems. Traditions are beliefs based on past practice or custom. Even today, many of our nursing practices, such as giving bed baths and taking vital signs at the beginning of the shift, are based on tradition.

Logical reasoning, which ancient Greek civilization employed to such advantage, provided a mental tool for examining the universe and human behavior. Logic, which is basic to the scientific method, involves deductive and inductive reasoning. The Greek contribution to scientific thinking was primarily the use of deductive reasoning, that is, the development of logical answers or conclusions from reliable premises; thus, deductive reasoning goes from the general to the particular. Of course, in deductive reasoning a great deal depends on the soundness of the premise or generalization. Inductive reasoning explains relationships by obtaining facts through observation and making generalizations based on these facts; thus, inductive reasoning goes from the particular to the general.

Scientific method, or research as we know it today, has been in use for a relatively short period of time, approximately 300 years. It makes use of logical reasoning; for example, the hypotheses to be tested by research, the methods of research used, and the conclusions reached as a result of research must always be logical.

Modern research, or scientific inquiry, may also make use of experts or authorities. Ideas or generalizations to be tested may be obtained from the experts as well as from practitioners. Scientific inquiry, however, provides a method whereby our ideas, hunches, or hypotheses can be systematically tested and valid evidence about the truth of the matter can be obtained. It rejects reliance on chance or magic, trial and error, or generalizations based on reasoning and experience alone.

RESEARCH IN NURSING

Because nursing is a practice profession, nurses have in the past placed more emphasis on its practical aspects than on research. Thus, nurses have tended to accept ideas and knowledge from authorities without much question.

Unlike many other professions, nursing was slow to develop the partnership between practitioner and investigator that is so necessary to achieve progress toward the ultimate goal—in this case, improved nursing care. There are several reasons for this situation. First, despite her skill in scientific investigation, Florence Nightingale laid the foundation for modern nursing education within the framework of the military tradition, which emphasizes the concept of authority. Schools of nursing that developed in hospitals throughout the world, including the United States, were strongly influenced by the British pattern of nursing education and thus continued to foster reliance on tradition and authority. It is interesting to speculate what might have happened had Miss Nightingale encouraged the spirit of inquiry in nursing as she did in other fields. The irony is that Miss Nightingale was an excellent statistician who made order out of a complex array of data. This belies the premise that nurses necessarily have an inbred fear of statistical research. Instead, nurses learn to use statistics as a means to an end—better care—not as an end in itself (Duffy, 1988).

In a discussion of the development of research in nursing, Simmons and Henderson (1964, p. 7) pointed out that the development of research within the established professions and the wealth of knowledge these professions have generated in the brief time that modern research methods have been used are directly related to the development of formal education within the university, a setting that serves as a center for research and research training. These authors suggest that it was necessary for nursing education programs to be established within universities before nurses could be prepared to do research. They also pointed to the fact that nursing education was influenced by the general status of all women in this country and by the educational facilities available to women prior to the turn of the century. University education for women then was certainly far from the common occurrence it is today.

As noted before, only recently in our history has nursing education been well established within colleges and universities. Although there were a few of these programs in the early part of this century, the major development of baccalaureate education for nurses did not begin until the latter half of the century. Hospital diploma education declined slowly as baccalaureate and associate degree programs grew, and admissions to baccalaureate programs exceeded those to hospital programs for the first time during the 1972 to 1973 school year (Johnson, 1977, p. 588).

At the 1982 American Nurses' Association (ANA) Biennial Convention, the ANA adopted the baccalaureate as the "minimum educational qualification for entry into professional nursing practice" (ANA Votes Federation, 1982, p. 1251). Recognizing the expanded opportunities for baccalaureate-prepared nurses, registered nurses (RNs) began returning to school in increasing numbers to earn the bachelor of science in nursing (BSN) degree. The number of RNs (with associate degrees or hospital diplomas) graduating from BSN programs rose from approximately 3,700 a year to more than 11,000 annually between 1975 and 1997 (American Association of Colleges of Nursing, 1997). In 1995, the Pew Health Professions Commission called for the closing of up to 20% of the nation's associate degree and hospital diploma nursing education programs in favor of accelerated support of baccalaureate and graduate degree nurse training (Pew Health Professions Commission, 1995).

Enrollment of master's degree students at U.S. nursing schools also rose in 1997 by 1.6% above the previous year, continuing a steady climb that has seen enrollments in master's nursing programs increase in 9 of the past 10 years (American Association of Colleges of Nursing, 1997). Continued growth is expected in master's education based on the demand for cost-effective, patient-focused caregivers. With the increase in baccalaureate and graduate education, more nurses than ever are obtaining preparation in research methods earlier in their professional careers. The National League for Nursing (1991) made critical thinking essential for its required accreditation outcome criteria, reflecting students' skills in reasoning, analyzing research, or decision making relevant to the discipline of nursing. Professional development and scholarship are outcomes associated with research and dissemination of knowledge through publications, presentations, media, technology, or grant writing by a program's students, faculty, and professional staff. Today it is a given that an understanding and appreciation of research is a prime ingredient of nursing practice and scholarship, and it bodes well for the future of the profession.

EARLY DAYS OF NURSING RESEARCH IN THE UNITED STATES

As nursing developed in this country, leadership resided primarily with the educators, who operated under the strong belief that nursing practice would be improved through improvement in the quality of nursing education. This thesis was logical in light of the status of nursing education, which was primarily an apprenticeship, and the status of education of women generally. These nursing educators were often responsible not only for the administration of the school but also for the nursing service. As a result, during the first half of the 20th century, research in nursing in the United States was directed more toward improved education or nursing service administration than toward improved practice.

Lillian Wald's Henry Street "experiment" and her school nursing demonstration project in New York City were early examples of nursing service projects aimed at improving health care (Dock, 1902; Schlotfeldt, 1977, p. 5; Wald, 1915). M. Adelaide Nutting's survey of nursing education, published in 1907, was probably the earliest important study in nursing education done by an American nurse. A few studies by nurses aimed at improving nursing care appeared in the literature in the 1920s and 1930s. These nurse authors were most often concerned with studies of nursing procedures or with time studies. For example,

Broadhurst, Rang, and Schoening (1927) studied hand brushing; Wasserberg and Northam (1927) did a time study in obstetrical nursing; Cowan (1929) carried out a comparative study of two methods of breast care; Pfefferkorn (1932) described time studies; Ryan and Miller (1932) did a thermometer study; and Wheeler (1938) reported on her study of tuberculosis nursing care.

Of considerable influence in promoting nursing studies during this period were such persons as Isabel Stewart and Mary M. Marvin (McManus, 1962). In 1927, Marvin made a plea in the *American Journal of Nursing* for nursing experimentation. She stated that there were

> six phases of experimentation which would help us in developing practical nursing along safer, sounder lines: First, an exhaustive study of nursing procedures from the standpoint of the biological and physical sciences; second, an analysis of nursing procedures on the basis of elimination of waste in materials, cost, energy, etc.; third, a comparative study of all equipment and materials used in the care of the sick; fourth, experimentation to find better methods of teaching the subject; fifth, tests for vocational aptitudes before the students enter the school; and sixth, tests of nursing performance, to determine the skill attained at any stage of teaching. (Marvin, 1927, pp. 331–332)

As we can see, half of her suggestions focused on studies of nursing procedures; the others were related to educational research. Nevertheless, interest in clinically oriented research was beginning to appear, although few nurses at that time were qualified to do research. Nursing research done in the 1930s and 1940s was frequently carried out by persons from other disciplines, such as education and sociology. Two well-known examples of such studies are Esther Lucille Brown's *Nursing for the Future* (1948) and *A Program for the Nursing Profession* by the Committee on the Function of Nursing (1948), chaired by Eli Ginsberg.

ACTIVITIES THAT INFLUENCE THE DEVELOPMENT OF NURSING RESEARCH

Research as a major movement in nursing received its first effective impetus in the 1950s. As a result of the recommendations of the Brown (1948) and Bridgman (1953) studies, among other developments, emphasis on baccalaureate and graduate education for nurses increased. Masters programs for nurses were developing, and a growing number of nurses were going on for the doctoral degree.

Some of the activities that influenced the development of nursing research were as follows:

1. In 1950, The House of Delegates of the ANA voted to initiate a nationwide program of studies of nursing functions. In May 1956, the ANA reported that during the 5-year project, a total of $400,000 was invested by nurses in this research, the purpose of which was to determine what nurses' functions should be and how to achieve better patient care despite personnel shortages. The researchers were looking for solid facts useful in future planning for education and service in nursing. Several state and local nursing groups were involved in the program, which was reported in *Nurses Invest in Patient Care* (American Nurses' Association Council of Nurse Researchers [ANACNR], 1956) and in *Twenty Thousand Nurses Tell Their Story* (Hughes, Hughes, & Deutscher, 1958).

2. In 1952, through the efforts of the Association of Collegiate Schools of Nursing, which became part of the National League for Nursing in that same year (Biennial highlights, pp. 824–825), the American Journal of Nursing Company began the publication of *Nursing Research.* The purposes of the new journal were "To inform members of the nursing profession and allied professions of the results of scientific studies in nursing, and to stimulate research in nursing" (A cooperative venture, *Nursing Research,* 1952, p. 5).

3. The Institute of Research and Service in Nursing Education was launched in 1953 at Teachers College, Columbia University (Bunge, 1958), to strengthen and improve education for nursing by conducting research on nursing and nursing education problems and disseminating the results and by preparing nurses to do research.

4. The ANA established the American Nurses' Foundation in 1955 as an independent organization for the purpose of furthering research in nursing by conducting and supporting research projects (Hardin, 1957; Taylor, 1970).

5. A Research Grant and Fellowship Branch was set up within the Division of Nursing Resources of the U.S. Public Health Service in 1955. Since its establishment, funds have been available for research in nursing, workshops and conferences, faculty development in research methods, fellowships, and nurse scientist training programs (Abdellah, 1970; Vreeland, 1964).

6. In 1957, a Department of Nursing was established within the Walter Reed Army Institute (Werley, 1962). Other federal agencies now have research programs in nursing.

7. In 1958, the House of Delegates of the ANA accepted Goal One, which was designed to stimulate nurses and other specialists to identify nursing principles and to do research on the application of these principles (ANACNR, 1960, p. 146). The Association's Committee on Research and Studies was given responsibility for planning activities

related to this research goal. They recognized two main activities: development of a corps of nurse researchers and development of intellectual curiosity and critical inquiry in students and in nurse practitioners (ANACNR, 1960). A conference group for nurses qualified in research was formed at the 1958 convention.

8. At the ANA's 1966 convention, one of the structural changes made was through the establishment of commissions. At its 1970 convention, the Commission on Nursing Research was established; in 1972, a Council of Nurse Researchers accountable to this commission was launched (Notter & Spalding, 1976, p. 331; See, 1977, p. 170).

Throughout the period from 1950 through 1972, nursing continued to be studied mostly by persons outside the profession. Nurses became one of the most frequently studied occupational groups—chiefly by behavioral scientists—but the study of nursing practice was still largely neglected. By 1959, however, the number of nurses with doctoral degrees reached 151 (Simmons & Henderson, 1964, p. 135), and the number of studies by nurses reported in the literature provided evidence of increased emphasis on research in nursing. Nursing education, however, remained the focus of many studies conducted by nurses at this time. The real impetus for research in clinical practice began in the 1960s. Gradually, interest in clinical investigations reported by nurses increased. Often these reports were based on doctoral studies, masters theses, or even occasionally on undergraduate work. Clinical research continued to lag behind other types of studies, however, even though 19 of the 72 articles published by *Nursing Research* in 1969 were related to nursing practice (Notter, 1970).

It was most encouraging that, in the "Editor's Report" in the January–February 1977 issue of *Nursing Research,* it was noted that clinical research reports represented nearly half of the previous year's contents (Carnegie, 1977). The May–June issue of the same year gave an excellent overview of clinical research; in fact, all of this 25th anniversary issue provided an interesting historical perspective on nursing research at that point. Stevenson (1987) provided another comprehensive guided tour of 35 years of nursing research in "Forging a Research Discipline." Brown, Tanner, and Padrick (1984) noted that by 1984 journals disseminating research had increased, with a shift away from acute illness toward prevention and health promotion. Furthermore, research had become more sophisticated and theoretically oriented. The need to develop instruments as well as to do replication studies continued.

During the 1970s a major issue in nursing centered around the development of models, conceptual frameworks, and theories to guide nursing practice. Another issue was the value of establishing a classification system for nursing diagnoses, and, in 1973, the North American Nursing Diagnoses Association (NANDA) published its first list of nursing diagnoses (Carpenito, 1984). The need for a formal taxonomy of nursing diagnoses and clinical validation through research became a continuing prerequisite for the 1980s.

Dissemination of research findings also became a priority in the 1970s and 1980s. A number of research journals were established during this time, including *Research in Nursing and Health, Advances in Nursing Science, Western Journal of Nursing Research, Scholarly Inquiry for Nursing Practice,* and *Applied Nursing Research. The Annual Review of Nursing Research,* launched by Werley and Fitzpatrick in 1983, signaled that the quantity of nursing research was sufficient that critical reviews of work in specific problem or topic areas were feasible (Stevenson, 1987).

The ANA Council of Nurse Researchers (ANACNR) held its first national research conference in 1973 and its first international research conference in 1987 in Washington, DC. Subsequent international conferences were held in Chicago, 1989; Los Angeles, 1991; and Washington, DC, 1993, 1996. Sigma Theta Tau, the international honor society of nursing, held its first international research conference in Madrid, Spain, in 1983, with subsequent international research conferences in Seoul, Korea, 1984; Tel Aviv, Israel, 1985; Edinburgh, Scotland, 1987; Taipei, Taiwan, 1989; Madrid, Spain, 1993; Sydney, Australia, 1994; Ocho Rios, Jamaica, 1996; Vancouver, British Columbia, 1997; Utrecht, The Netherlands, 1998; and London, England, 1999. The number of research conferences increased during the 1970s and 1980s, and they continue to influence nursing research development. Stevenson (1987, p. 63) wrote, "Personal stories imply that many nurses were inspired to complete graduate programs, write grant applications, redo their data analyses, or publish research findings as a result of advice and inspiration experienced in the research conference milieu."

In 1985, the ANA Cabinet on Research issued *Directions for Nursing Research: Toward the 21st Century* (ANACNR, 1985). The priorities were based on their stated goal for nurses doing research, scientifically based knowledge useful to nursing practice. Examples of clinical research related to the priorities are listed (ANACNR, 1985). The Council of Nurse Researchers published a revised copy of *Directions* in 1993 (ANACNR, 1993).

Throughout the 1980s, emphasis continued to be on good clinical research, but it was also recognized by many that there must be a balance in the kinds of research related to nursing. Although clinical studies receive priority for the purpose of improvement of patient care, investigation of methods of providing nursing service, nursing education studies, and philosophical and historical research is required for nursing to obtain the broad base of verified facts it needs to develop a body of scientific knowledge. Another important priority is reiterated here: the need to develop instruments appropriate to the study of nursing practice variables and to test these instruments adequately (see Ventura, Hinshaw, & Atwood, 1981).

In 1987 the ANA Cabinet on Nursing Research and the Council of Nurse Researchers, through the editorial efforts of their former elected members Jacqueline Clinton and Kathleen A. McCormick, distributed a brochure, *Research in Nursing: Toward a Science in Nursing*, to legislators and the lay public (ANACNR, 1987). The brochure described the benefits of nursing research for the health of the American people and discussed issues that legislators and consumers need to know about nursing research to support allocation of funds and resources for its development (Hott, 1987). It has been available through Publications Orders (D-52), ANA Publications.

In 1985, following up on the recommendations of the Institute of Medicine study from 2 years prior, Congress moved nursing research to the mainstream of scientific research when it authorized the National Center for Nursing Research (NCNR) as a provision of the National Institutes of Health (NIH) reauthorization bill (Public Law 99-158, the Health Research Extension Act of 1985; see Bauknecht, 1985). A change in status of the center to an institute received positive federal legislative and administrative review, and in 1993 the NCNR became the National Institute of Nursing Research (NINR). Doris Merritt, M.D., was the NCNR's first acting director (Merritt, 1986) until the formal appointment of a nurse researcher as director, Ada Sue Hinshaw, R.N., Ph.D., in May 1987. Patricia A. Grady, R.N., Ph.D., became nurse director in 1996.

As the focal point of the nation's nursing research activities, the NINR supports clinical and basic research to establish a scientific basis for the care of individuals across the life span, from management of patients during illness and recovery to the reduction of risks for disease and disability and the promotion of healthy lifestyles (National Institute of Nursing Research, 1998). Opportunities for funding identified by the NINR can be categorized according to three major themes (Grady, 1998): (1) Chronic Illnesses or Conditions, represented by symptom management of chronic neurological conditions, rehabilitation issues in traumatic brain injury, and improvement of quality of life for transplantation patients; (2) Behavioral Changes and Interventions, consisting of research into extending advances in cardiovascular risk factor management to special populations; and (3) Responding to Compelling Health Concerns, with an emphasis on end-of-life care. In addition to encouraging high-quality nursing research, the NINR provides leadership to expand the pool of experienced nurse researchers through comprehensive research training programs. These programs prepare individuals with the requisite interdisciplinary skills to conduct nursing research, thus helping to ensure that there will be an adequate cadre of well-trained nurse scientists to meet the nursing research needs of the future. The NINR also serves as a base for interaction with other areas of health care research. Through its collaboration with other NIH components, nursing research expands the information base and therapeutic potency not only of nursing but also of all health disciplines. The brightest discoveries come when research questions are viewed from different perspectives. With the establishment of the NINR, nursing research was put on an equal level with the health research community because science produced by nurses is critiqued by other health care disciplines. For updated reports on activities of the NINR see "News from NINR," a regularly appearing column in *Nursing Outlook* (Grady, 1997).

According to the ANA Standards of Clinical Nursing Practice (1997) it is the responsibility of all practicing nurses to use research findings in practice. Nurses are expected to use interventions substantiated by research. The nurse is also expected to participate in research activities as appropriate to the individual's position, education, and practice environment. Today, preparation in research methods is an integral part of education at all levels of professional nursing. At the baccalaureate level, an introduction to research with an emphasis on using research findings in practice prepares nurses to be critical consumers of research. Nurses prepared with baccalaureate and higher degrees in nursing must be able to read, comprehend, analyze, and evaluate the scientific merits of research reports in order to draw conclusions about the usefulness of new knowledge and participate in developing research-based practice protocols and guidelines (Barnsteiner, 1997). At the master's level, nurses are prepared to be active members of research teams. Master's-prepared nurses are able to assume the role of clinical expert collaborating with experienced investigators in proposal development, data collection, data analysis, and interpretation. Doctoral education and postdoctoral education prepares nurses to contribute to nursing knowledge through the conduct of independently funded research projects (American Nurses Association, 1989; Davis & Burnard, 1992). The demand for doctorally prepared nurses continues. Although the number of awards of new nursing doctorates grew to 401 in 1995, the increase occurred at an average of 9 additional graduates in each of the previous 5 years, a snail's pace that educators say is far below the rate needed to expand nursing's research base to address a growing list of contemporary health problems (American Association of Colleges of Nursing, 1996).

It is estimated that by the year 2000, the demand for nurses prepared to function in advanced practice clinical specialties, teaching, and research is expected to outstrip the supply significantly. According to the *American Association of Colleges of Nursing Media Backgrounder* (December, 1997), in 1996 only about 9% and 0.6% of employed RNs held a masters or doctoral degree, respectively, as their highest educational preparation. The number of doctoral programs in nursing in U.S. universities grew from 14 in 1977 to 38 in 1987 and to 62 in 1997. Moreover, nursing schools reported plans to develop 17 additional doctoral programs (American Association of Colleges of Nursing, 1997). Increased numbers of programs do not ensure quality, however, and both the American Association of Colleges of Nursing (AACN) and the National League for Nursing (NLN) have noted the need for a careful look at evaluating doctoral programs in order to promote and ensure that our future nurse scientists are adequately prepared to meet our research mission. Commenting on doctoral preparation, Lynaugh (1997) notes, "For the first time in their history, nurses are able, because of their doctoral training, and their position and experiences as scholars and researchers, to compete on the same grounds as researchers in biomedicine, health services, and other fields" (p. 14).

We make progress slowly, but as a true partnership develops between researcher and practitioner, nurses will move closer to their common goal—the achievement of better care for patients, care that is based on validated scientific inquiry.

NURSING RESEARCH NOW AND IN THE FUTURE

The current status and future of nursing research are promising and challenging. The challenge is not only to have the value of nursing research acknowledged but also to forge new directions that further develop and define the databases that show nurses' role in health care delivery as well as health outcomes that demonstrate the effectiveness of nursing care. The central goal of nursing research is to find answers to important clinical questions and to put that knowledge to practical use (Dexter, 1997). Nursing's research agenda needs to focus on health promotion, health care systems, and carefully articulated outcomes (Sigma Theta Tau International, 1996). New directions for nursing research in the 21st century identify the need for studies that focus on a health care policy emphasizing treatment quality and cost effectiveness; the movement toward managed care systems that focus on primary care, health promotion, and disease prevention; effective management of acute and chronic illnesses; the growth of health care technology; and ongoing interest in quality of life issues (Pollner, 1997). A number of promising new models of health care provision and community health promotion that are consistent with the restructured health care system and nursing roles either exist or are being developed (Sigma Theta Tau International, 1996). Many universities have established nursing research centers where a number of nurse scientists work together on advancing programs of research. For example, the Frances Payne Bolton School of Nursing at Case Western Reserve, the University of California San Francisco, Indiana University, the University of Pennsylvania, and the University of Washington have large funded nursing research centers. Some of the ongoing programs of research at these centers focus on the needs of the chronically ill, elders, women, and children and on improving health care delivery to vulnerable groups during a time of dramatic shifts in the sites of health care (Nagelkerk, Henry, & Brooten, 1997). Also, some academic and clinical research centers have initiated the practice of publishing comprehensive newsletters reporting their activities. These newsletters are shared with other interested nursing research groups and individuals. Examples of newsletters currently in circulation include "Pulse," a joint publication of the Indiana University School of Nursing and the Indiana University School of Nursing Alumni Association; "The Science of Caring," published by the School of Nursing and Nursing Alumni Association of the University of California San Francisco; "The Stanford Nurse," published by Stanford Health Services, Stanford University; "Vital Signs," published by the University of Illinois at Chicago; and "The Beth Israel Nurse," published by Beth Israel Medical Center, New York.

Today, there is increased opportunity for networking through regional, national, and international nursing research conferences, and journals. International nursing research conferences, such as those sponsored by ANA Council of Nurse Researchers, Sigma Theta Tau, and International Council of Nurses (ICN), draw increased numbers of nurse researchers who present and participate in research sessions. Sigma Theta Tau International also sponsors regional and local research conferences. Regional nursing research conferences such as those of the Midwest Regional Nursing Society (MRNS), Western Institute of Nursing (WIN), Western Society of Research in Nursing (WSRN), Southern Nursing Research Society (SNRS), and Eastern Nursing Research Society (ENRS) that resulted from the merging of the New England Organization of Nursing (NEON) and the Mid-Atlantic Regional Nursing Association (MARNA) are well attended. Specialty organizations, such as the Association for Women's Health, Obstetric and Neonatal Nurses (AWHONN), Oncology Nursing Society (ONS), American Association of Critical Care Nurses (AACN), and the Society of Pediatric Nurses (SPN), also hold regional research conferences that facilitate networking. A potential benefit of networking with other nurse researchers in the same approximate geographic area who have similar research interest is the opportunity to collaborate in research and to pool knowledge and resources. In a newsletter column about the 1997 ENRS Conference in Philadelphia, McDonald (1998) provided an excellent illustration of this point:

> During a session on pain management, April Hazard Vallerand presented her research on the "Development of an Instrument of Measure Functional Status in Women with Chronic Pain." During the same session, Rhea Sanford and Terese Donovan presented research that they and their clinical nurse specialist colleagues had conducted, "Educational Interventions and Their Effects on Nurse's Knowledge Regarding Pain." Following the session the three began to discuss the issue of strengthening pain management knowledge for nurses in acute settings. Dr. Vallerand had begun some pain management consulting in an acute care setting, and was interested in the vignettes developed and used during the pain management education intervention. The vignettes were graciously shared, and help illustrate the valuable collaboration that happen through ENRS. (pp. 5–6)

Pooling resources and collaboration may also help to overcome problems associated with small samples so common in nursing research due to lack of funds because research grants are so competitive.

As the world continues to get smaller through the use of information technology such as electronic mail, facsimile machines, the Internet, and video conferencing, we can predict not only more international conferences and collaboration but also more cross-cultural studies as well. Farrell, Farrell, and Jogenson (1990) have written about how a European network can be developed to become a potential hub for such a global nursing system. Making nursing research ethnically and culturally relevant will become even more significant as the world becomes a global village (National Association of the American College of Obstetrics and Gynecology, 1991). (See chapter 10 for more on computers in research.)

The future of research in nursing and nursing research depends on your knowledge of the art and science of clinical nursing practice, and its "dailiness." As Wilson (1991, p. 282) whimsically describes it, quoting Alice Walker, author of *The Color Purple,* "The act of knowing from our own experience is so simple that many of us have spent years discovering it. We have constantly looked high when we should have looked high and low." Wilson says, "It has been said of conducting research that, like Wagner's music, it is better than it sounds" (p. 282). Perhaps we need to put more light on both Wagner and research as a sensory experience to catch the excitement of nursing research! You hold the future in your intellectual curiosity, commitment, and professional skill. It is essential that nurses communicate to consumers and policy makers what it is that nursing does that is newsworthy and informative so that all of us can benefit in knowing what our research is all about (Wakefield, 1998). Hinshaw (1989) predicts that in the future research will be an acknowledged way of life for all professionals. It is interesting to note that nursing is not the only health profession struggling to link practice and research. Medicine is going through a similar soul searching, and proponents of a new technique of medical decision making called "evidence-based medicine" think they have finally solved this problem (Zuger, 1997). Evidence-based practice involves trying whenever possible to base medical decisions on sound research data, rather than relying on a combination of habit and casual intuition, using tests and treatments that they are familiar with or that seem to work. Our physician friends, too, are recognizing "there's a science to the art of medicine."

Hinshaw (1992) emphasizes the need to weave together the biological and social in doing nursing research. As convention keynoter for the New York State Nurses Association, Hinshaw said "Research is the key to excellence" (p. 4). You can light up your practice, your professional life, and nursing's future with nursing research (Feldman & Hott, 1991).

REFERENCES

Abdellah, F. G. (1970). Overview of nursing research 1955–1968. Part I, *Nursing Research, 19,* 6–17; Part II, *Nursing Research, 19,* 151–162; Part III, *Nursing Research, 19,* 239–252.

American Association of Colleges of Nursing. (1996, July). *Nursing schools seek balance of teaching and research skills in effort to boost the Ph.D. supply.* (AACN Issue Bulletin). Washington, DC: Author.

American Association of Colleges of Nursing. (1997, December). *Nursing school enrollments: Some vital perspectives.* (AACN Media Backgrounder). Washington, DC: Author.

American Association of Colleges of Nursing. (1997). 1997–1998 *Enrollment and graduations in baccalaureate and graduate programs in nursing.* Washington, DC: Author.

American Nurses Association. (1989). *Education for participation in nursing research.* Kansas City, MO: Author.

American Nurses Association. (1997). *Standards of clinical nursing practice.* Washington, DC: Author.

American Nurses Association Council of Nurse Researchers. (1956). *Nurses invest in patient care.* New York: American Nurses Association.

American Nurses Association Council of Nurse Researchers. (1960). House of Delegates reports, 1958–1960. New York: American Nurses Association.

American Nurses Association Council of Nurse Researchers. (1985). *Directions for nursing research: Toward the 21st century.* Kansas City, MO: American Nurses Association.

American Nurses Association Council of Nurse Researchers. (1993). *Directions for nursing research.* Washington, DC: Author.

American Nurses Association Council of Nurse Researchers. (1987). *Research in nursing: Toward a science in nursing.* Kansas City, MO: American Nurses Association.

American Nurses Association Votes Federation. (1982). *American Journal of Nursing, 82,* 1251.

Barnsteiner, J. (1997). New directions for nursing inquiry. *Penn Nursing, 2*(1), 18–21.

Bauknecht, V. (1985). Capital Commentary: NIH Bill passes, includes nursing research center. *American Nurse, 17*(10), 2.

Biennial highlights. (1952). *American Journal of Nursing, 52,* 824–827.

Bridgman, M. (1953). *Collegiate Education for Nursing.* New York: Russell Sage Foundation.

Broadhurst, J., Rang, G. G., & Schoening, E. (1927). Hand brush suggestions for visiting nurses. *Public Health Nursing, 19,* 487–489.

Brown, E. L. (1948). *Nursing for the future.* New York: Russell Sage Foundation.

Brown, J. S., Tanner, C. A., & Padrick, K. (1984). Nursing's search for scientific knowledge. *Nursing Research, 33,* 26–32.

Bunge, H. L. (1958). The Institute of Research and Service in Nursing Education, Teachers College, Columbia University. *Nursing Research, 7,* 113–115.

Carnegie, M. E. (1977). Editor's report—1977 [Editorial]. *Nursing Research, 26,* E3.

Carpenito, L. J. (1984). *Handbook of nursing diagnosis.* Philadelphia: Lippincott.

Committee on the Function of Nursing. (1948). In E. Ginsberg (Chairman), *A program for the nursing profession.* New York: Macmillan.

A cooperative venture. (1952).[Editorial]. *Nursing Research, 1,* 5.

Cowan, C. M. (1929). A study of breast care. Part I, *American Journal of Nursing, 29,* 1165–1170; Part II, *American Journal of Nursing, 29,* 1299–1306.

Davis, B., & Burnard, P. (1992). Academic levels in nursing. *Journal of Advanced Nursing, 17* (12), 1395–1400.

Dexter, P. (1997, Spring). Nurse researchers build on prior studies to find answers to important clinical questions. *Pulse* (A joint publication of the Indiana University School of Nursing and the Indiana University School of Nursing Alumni Association). pp. 9–12.

Dock, L. L. (1902). School nurse experiment in New York. *American Journal of Nursing,* 3, 108–110.

Duffy, M. E. (1988). Statistics: Friend or foe? *Nursing and Health Care, 9,* 73-75.

Farrell, M., Farrell, J., & Jogenson, I. V. (1990). A European and global strategy for a nursing information network. *International Nursing Review, 37,* 271–279.

Feldman, H. R., & Hott, J. R. (1991). Light up your practice with nursing research. *Journal of the New York State Nurses Association, 22,* 8–11.

Grady, P. (1997). News from NINR, *Nursing Outlook, 45*(2), 72.

Grady, P. (1998). News from NINR, *Nursing Outlook, 46*(1), 43.

Hardin, C. (1957). The American Nurses' Foundation builds a program. *American Journal of Nursing, 57,* 310–311.

Hinshaw, A. (1989). Nursing science: The challenge to develop knowledge. *Nursing Science Quarterly, 2,* 162–171.

Hinshaw, A. S. (1992). Keynote speaker invites every RN to participate in nursing research. *Report of the New York State Nurses Association, 23*(10), 4.

Hott, J. R. (1987, June). Message from the chairperson. *ANA Council's Annual Report Newsletter,* 16–17.

Hughes, E. C., Hughes, H. MacG., & Deutscher, I. (1958). *Twenty thousand nurses tell their story.* Philadelphia: Lippincott.

Johnson, W. L. (1977). Educational preparation for nursing—1976. *Nursing Outlook, 25,* 587–592.

Lynaugh, J. (1997). Mainstreaming nursing research. *Penn Nursing, 2*(1), 14.

Marvin, M. M. (1927). Research in nursing. *American Journal of Nursing, 27,* 331–335.

McDonald, D. (1998, Winter). Membership in ENRS promotes collaboration. *Newsletter of the Eastern Nursing Research Society,* 4–5.

McManus, R. L. (1962). Isabel M. Stewart—Foremost researcher. *Nursing Research, 11,* 4, 6.

Merritt, D. M. (1986). The National Center for Nursing Research. *Image, 18,* 84–85.

Nagelkerk, J., Henry, S., & Brooten, D. (1997). Commentary about Martinson's nursing research: Obstacles and challenges. *Image: Journal of Nursing Scholarship, 29*(4), 324.

National Institute of Nursing Research. (1998, January 14). *Web Updates: NINR Mission* [On-line]. Available: http://www.nih.gov/ninr/NINRMission.htm/.

National League for Nursing. (1991). *Interpretive guidelines for standards and criteria, accrediting commission.* New York: Author.

Notter, L. E. (1970). Report of the editor—1970 [Editorial]. *Nursing Research, 19,* 5.

Notter, L. E., & Spalding, E. K. (1976). *Professional nursing: Foundations, perspectives, and relationships* (9th ed.). Philadelphia: Lippincott.

Nurses Association of the American College of Obstetrics and Gynecology. (1991). Making nursing research culturally relevant. *Women's Health Nursing Scan,* 5, 1–2.

Nursing Research (1977). 25th Anniversary Issue, *26,* 163–227.

Nutting, M. A. (1907). The education and professional position of nurses. In *Report of the Commissioner of Education for the Year Ending June 30, 1906* (pp. 155–205). Washington, DC: U.S. Government Printing Office.

Pew Health Professions Commission. (1995, November). *Critical challenges: Revitalizing the health professions for the twenty-first century* (p. 51). San Francisco: University of California-San Francisco, Center for the Health Professions.

Pfefferkorn, B. (1932). Measuring nursing, quantitatively and qualitatively. *American Journal of Nursing, 32,* 80–84.

Pollner, F. (1997). Nursing research: New directions for the 21st century. *NIH Catalyst, 5*(1).

Ryan, E., & Miller, V. B. (1932). Disinfection of clinical thermometers. *American Journal of Nursing, 32,* 197–206.

Schlotfeldt, R. M. (1977). Nursing research: Reflections of values. *Nursing Research, 26,* 4–9.

See, E. M. (1977). The ANA and research in nursing. *Nursing Research, 26,* 165–171.

Sigma Theta Tau International. (1996). *Arista II: A synopsis of actions and recommendations for the preferred future of nursing.* Indianapolis: Author.

Simmons, L. W., & Henderson, V. (1964). *Nursing research: A survey and assessment.* New York: Appleton-Century-Crofts.

Sinclair, V. G. (1987). Literature searches by computer. *Image, 19,* 35–37.

Stevenson, J. S. (1987). Forging a research discipline. *Nursing Research, 36,* 60–63.

Taylor, S. D. (1970). American Nurses' Foundation, 1955–1970. *Nursing Research Report, 5,* 1–6.

Ventura, M. R., Hinshaw, A. S., & Atwood, J. R. (1981). Instrumentation: The next step [Editorial]. *Nursing Research, 30,* 257.

Vreeland, E. M. (1964). Nursing research programs of the Public Health Service: Highlights and trends. *Nursing Research, 13,* 148–158.

Wakefield, M. K. (1998). *National panel begins dialogue on nursing. Nursing Excellence: Special Post-conference issue.* Indianapolis, IN: Sigma Theta Tau International.

Wald, L. D. (1915). *House on Henry Street.* New York: Holt.

Wasserberg, C., & Northam, E. (1927). Some time studies in obstetrical nursing. *American Journal of Nursing, 27,* 543–544.

Werley, H. H. (1962). Promoting the research dimension in the practice of nursing through the establishment and development of a Department of Nursing in an Institute of Research. *Military Medicine, 127,* 219–231.

Wheeler, C. A. (ed.). (1938). A study of the nursing care of tuberculosis patients. *American Journal of Nursing, 38,* 1021–1037.

Wilson, H. S. (1991). Identifying problems for clinical research to create a nursing tapestry. *Nursing Outlook, 39,* 280–282.

Zuger, A. (1997, December 16). New way of doctoring: By the book. *New York Times,* F 1–7.

2

The Meaning and Purpose of Research

Why research? Particularly, why research in nursing? Scientific investigations can be long and costly and may end up with negative findings. Research, however, some of which did not at the time appear to have immediate practical value, has been responsible for most of the major advances our society has made in the last century—advances in communication technology, transportation, agriculture, genetic engineering, and the control and treatment of disease, to mention but a few. Modern electronic technology is a direct product of research. Modern medical treatment had its origin in various types of chemical and biological research, both basic and applied. Such simple, taken-for-granted things as refrigeration, air-conditioning, radio, television, and computers all came about as a result of the investigations by many scientists. It is easy to see the importance of research in our lives if we but stop and think about it for a moment.

What about research in nursing? Is it really needed? Is it really important? In the past, nursing relied heavily on facts and knowledge obtained from authorities, that is, facts and knowledge derived from the experience of experts. It also borrowed facts from other sciences without necessarily testing them scientifically to determine how well they might serve in their new role.

Modern research methods are tools that nurses can employ in studying our practice to obtain scientific evidence needed for validating that practice and for using the findings of our investigations in our practice. Because these methods are known, it would seem that all nurses are morally responsible to use them for the improvement of patient care.

WAYS OF PARTICIPATING IN RESEARCH

You, as a nurse, can participate in research in several ways. First, you can observe nursing care that is being given and the responses of patients to that care. Because the clinical area is rich with problems that you can translate into research projects, you can raise questions that should be studied. For example, Budin (1998) noted in the literature and in her practice in women's health that married women with supportive partners seemed to adjust reasonably well to breast cancer; little was known, however, about the impact of breast cancer among women who were single, divorced or separated, or widowed. Her observations led to her interest in studying factors related to psychosocial adjustment to breast cancer in unmarried women. The findings identified social support and symptom distress as two important factors related to psychosocial adjustment to breast cancer in these unmarried women. Type of surgery was not a factor related to adjustment. Implications for health care providers to facilitate positive psychosocial adjustment to breast cancer in unmarried women are suggested.

Fahs and Kinney (1991) noted that the abdomen was usually recommended as the preferred injection site for low-dose heparin therapy in hospitalized patients at risk for developing thrombophlebitis, even though the basis for this recommendation was not supported with empirical evidence. Because using the abdomen for injections may frighten the patient and inconvenience the nurse, Fahs and Kinney (1991) designed a study to determine whether the thigh and arm were effective as alternate sites in accomplishing the goal of low-dose heparin therapy and to identify any differences in bruising at the injection site. They found no significant differences among the three sites in activated partial thromboplastin time (APTT) or bruising, thus the clinical practice of using the abdomen as the only or preferred site for subcutaneous heparin injections was not supported.

In another instance, Schepp (1991) questioned what helps or hinders parents' ability to cope with their child's hospitalization at 1 to 24 months of age. Building on past research and a scientific rationale about coping, control, and anxiety, Schepp predicted that if mothers knew more about their child's condition they would feel they had more control over the situation. If they knew more about what to expect and felt more in control, Schepp speculated, their anxiety would be reduced, leaving more energy for them to cope with their child's hospitalization. Her interviews with 45 mothers of acutely ill children 2 to 7 days following admission showed that the mothers who did know what to expect reported less anxiety and used less effort to cope with this potentially traumatic experience. Nevertheless, perceived control did not appear to be influenced by the mother's knowledge, anxiety level, or coping effort. Feldman and Hott (1991) pointed out that single studies such as Schepp's (1991) could not necessarily be generalized to others but that the study's findings showed that a nurse could include nursing interventions, such as providing mothers with more information about expectations, to help mothers be more supportive in this stressful time.

Bookbinder (1992a, 1992b), whose doctoral thesis addresses nurses' use of research in clinical settings, describes the "dailiness" (Wilson, 1991) of nursing research when nurses ask questions and try to answer them. In this example, nurses at Memorial Sloan Kettering Cancer Center in New York asked why they needed to change intravenous (IV) tubing every 4 hours when it was changed every 48 or 72 hours in other institutions. Their question involved both patient care and cost-effectiveness issues. After identifying the problem and searching the literature about the incidence of increased susceptibility to infection when tubes are changed, they developed a proposal for their Nursing Quality Assurance (QA) Committee that eventually prompted a policy to change tubing every 72 hours and resulted in cost savings of more than $150,000 a year. As a result of your observations, you too may propose an exploratory study, or you may communicate your observations to a nurse researcher who may carry out the study or assist you in doing so. You might think about this and compile a list of observations you would like to make and some of the variables that would be involved.

A second way of participating in nursing research is to assist in the collection of data for a research project. As the amount of nursing research increases, so do the opportunities for nurses to become involved in research programs. Some researchers employ research assistants to help with such data collection procedures as making observations or conducting interviews. For the past 21 years, thousands of registered nurses (RNs) have participated as data collectors in the Nurses Health Study conducted by Frank Speizer, M.D., and a team of researchers at the Harvard Medical School. Some key findings of this research indicated that smoking, the dominant cause of lung cancer and heart disease in women, was also linked to cataracts, stroke, pancreatic cancer, and possibly colon cancer and that regular physical activity helps to keep weight down and protects against diabetes, heart disease, osteoporosis, and colon cancer. In this longitudinal study, nurses were found to be so reliable in the collection of data that Speizer and his team added 25,000 children of the second group of nurses included in the project. The new project, called "Growing up today," focused on weight concerns, physical activity, diet, growth and development, and generational health and well-being. This example clearly demonstrates that in addition to contributing to the care of patients in hospitals, clinics, schools, and homes, nurses also contribute to the future health of the nation through their dedication and enthusiastic participation in research (Forman, 1997).

Being a member of a research team, intradisciplinary or interdisciplinary, is another way of participating. The team may consist of all nurses: for example, "Social Support and Patterns of Adjustment to Breast Cancer" was carried out by a team consisting of an experienced nurse researcher, five doctoral students, a director of nursing research at a clinical agency, and a clinical nurse specialist in oncology (Hoskins et al., 1996).

The project described previously about the group of nurses who worked together concerning the frequency of changing IV tubing is another example of collaborative research by nurses (Bookbinder, 1992b). Rempusheski (1989) pointed out how clinical nurses gain by working on an established study with a nurse researcher, learning about the research process by doing it and creating a tailor-made experience to meet their individual learning objectives. Being involved in an investigation and then waiting to see how it turns out, knowing that you have contributed to the project, is an exciting experience.

You may be the only nurse on a clinical team headed by a sociologist, psychologist, physician, or physiologist. In this case, as the nursing expert, your clinical knowledge will be as important as your knowledge of study methods. Nurses are bringing their unique, valuable perspectives to interdisciplinary research teams studying health services in the United States at the Harvard Nursing Research Institute (Saver, 1998). This postdoctoral research program prepares nurses to have advanced expertise in research methods. According to director, Peter Buerhaus, R.N., Ph.D., "nurses study side-by-side with fellows from many other disciplines, including physicians, attorneys, managers, economist, biostatisticians, epidemiologists, and public health practitioners. This experience gives nurses, as well as their peers, a deeper understanding of complex health issues, and gives them the expertise to work collaboratively and effectively with a team" (Saver, 1998, pp. 6–7).

A number of intradisciplinary teams that included nurses have investigated the problems associated with the increased use of latex gloves, triggered in part by the AIDS epidemic. Studies suggest that as many as 10% of the nation's 2.2 million RNs suffer from latex allergy. Between January 1990 and June 1993, a study by the Department of Internal Medicine in Rochester, Minnesota, showed that 104 of 342 Mayo Medical Center employees who had symptoms of latex allergy tested positively for the allergy. Of these, 40 were nurses, mostly in general practice. Concerned by the increase in latex allergy among nurses, the ANA is working with the National Institute for Occupational Safety and Health and the Occupational Safety and Health Administration (OSHA) to deal with this problem (Marks, 1996).

Another example of interdisciplinary research involving nurses is the work of a task force convened by the National Institute of Child Health and Human Development (NICHD) (1997) of the NIH. This group, composed of representatives from medicine, nursing, epidemiology, basic science, and the public interest, worked to identify a nomenclature system for Electronic Fetal Monitoring (EFM) interpretation, a move that will provide a foundation for further clinical research that may improve the predictive value for EFM.

As a team member, you may also be responsible for carrying out an individual piece of research on your own while others on the team contribute other pieces. Working on a research team may be your first step to becoming a full-fledged researcher. Brooten was the nurse researcher or principal investigator of a clinical team made up of physicians, nurses, and others to investigate a research question dealing with early discharge of very low birth weight infants that was published in a prestigious medical journal, the *New England Journal of Medicine* (Brooten et al., 1986).

GETTING THE EXPERT HELP YOU NEED

Of course, a meaningful way of participating in nursing research is to conduct a study yourself. Although conducting research usually requires an advanced degree, this book presents some of the basic facts a researcher needs to know before even a simple study is attempted. In addition, a novice researcher may want to obtain help from an expert in research, such as a doctorally prepared faculty member or a consultant. Your institution may have on its staff a nurse qualified in research methods who is available to assist you. Perhaps your local university may be able to suggest a contact for you. Some institutions have established research centers for this purpose. For example, Molloy College's Department of Nursing's Center for Research and Scholarly Practice provides prospective nurse researchers with the support and guidance they need to transform ideas into research studies (Kramer, 1998). In this center, experienced researchers are willing to work alongside novices every step of the way. Support may also take the form of networking, in which researchers are introduced to other nurses with similar research interests. In addition to your local setting, your regional nursing society, Sigma Theta Tau International, or the American Academy of Nursing may, through their membership, suggest a contact for you. Organizations such as the ENRS (1998), the Society of Rogerian Scholars (1998), and state nurses associations (New York State Nurses Association [NYSNA], 1998) publish directories of nurse researchers and identify special research interests. Many conferences now provide special sessions for research consultation. For example, at the 1998 AWHONN National Convention individuals could register for a half-hour session of one-on-one consultation with expert nurse researchers to talk about an ongoing project, how to get started, funding sources, or getting published (Association for Women's Health, Obstetrics and Neonatal Nurses [AWHONN], 1998). You may need help to narrow your research problem down to one that is manageable for the study you have in mind. An expert can often also help by making suggestions about where to look for information or related reports in the literature. You will also probably look for guidance in locating or developing your research tool and in analyzing the data you collect. Do not expect to have your work done for you, however; that guidance will help you learn to do the research yourself.

Later, as a result of your interest and experience, you may undertake the graduate work required to become a fully qualified researcher. It is very important that more nurses obtain this type of preparation if nursing is to have the research leadership it needs. Despite the increased enrollments and graduations, the future demand for nurses with advanced degrees will exceed availability. By the year 2005, the estimated shortfall of master's and doctorally prepared nurses will stand at about 200,000 (U.S. Department of Health and Human Services, 1990). Hopefully, the laws of supply and demand will bode well for the nurse researcher.

BE CREATIVE AND REPLICATE

Development of nursing science requires not only new research, but also replication studies that repeat another exploration or procedure, allowing for increased confidence in the findings (Martin, 1995). Replication is defined as the repeat testing of the same relationship using a variety of studies that have evaluated the relationship with different samples (Feldman & Hott, 1991). Campbell, Poland, Waller, and Ager (1992) replicated several other retrospective studies with respect to determining the prevalence of prenatal partner assault and added assessment of assault by other persons during pregnancy. This study extended the literature on abuse during pregnancy by examining correlates of battering during pregnancy and the association between battering during pregnancy and adequacy of prenatal care. In another example, Rice, Mullin, and Jarosz (1992) partially replicated and extended an earlier study (Rice & Johnson, 1984) to compare the effects of two approaches to teaching postoperative therapeutic exercise (preadmission self-instruction and postadmission instruction by a nurse) on postadmission mood state, exercise performance, and teaching time and on postoperative recovery in patients having coronary artery bypass graft (CABG) surgery. Replication studies in nursing are essential to develop the substantive content needed for the professional discipline and to present appropriate research results to our clinicians, colleagues, and the public. Beck (1994) describes different replication strategies for nursing research and includes a comprehensive review of replication studies published in nursing journals from 1983 to 1992. It is interesting to note that in her review only 49 replication studies were found. Beck argues that implementing research findings into nursing practice has been seriously hampered by the lack of replication studies. She urges others to give it a try, stating "replication research is not simple, dull, and repetitive. It takes considerable imagination and skill. Through replication research, new directions in methodology and theory are found" (Beck, 1994, p. 191).

BECOME AN INFORMED CONSUMER

Suppose you do not wish to be actively involved in conducting research, or you do not have an opportunity to be involved. What then? You still have an important responsibility, one that in the long run justifies research. This is the responsibility of being an informed consumer of the findings of scientific inquiry. A consumer of research reads and evaluates reports of studies to keep up-to-date on information that might be relevant to his or her practice or to develop new skills. Bookbinder (1992c) reports on nurses who questioned standard practice in the postanesthesia care unit (PACU), where patients were lying flat despite their obvious discomfort and increased cough when supine for the pulmonary artery pressure (PAP) readings. In this case, the nurses sought out the scientific studies that supported leaving their patients' bodies elevated during the PAP readings and brought the results of their literature review to the central Nursing QA Committee. The procedure change was not only approved but also adopted by the physicians who had established the original policy the nurses had so wisely questioned.

USE RESEARCH-BASED PROTOCOLS

One of the oft-repeated laments of nurse researchers is that research findings do not find their way into the clinical practice of nurses (Feldman, Haber, & Hott, 1993). The belief has been expressed that there is a gap between knowledge verified by research and its use by the practitioner. In a national survey of nearly 1,000 clinical nurses, barriers that prevented nurses from being actively involved in research use included failure to find studies related to a problem, inability to understand research reports, insufficient time on the job to implement new ideas, and lack of authority to chance patient care procedures (Funk, Champagne, Wiese, & Tornquist, 1991). How can nurses become more active and discriminating consumers? First they need to acknowledge the historical and contemporary underuse of research findings to guide practice. Next they need to maximize usage opportunities that already exist within our organizations and develop innovative ways to increase our consumer behavior. For example, a group of nurses from a hospital in New Jersey read about a new nursing protocol enabling women's health care providers to screen routinely for urinary incontinence and volunteered to evaluate the protocol and provide women with information about incontinence (Elkind, 1998). The protocol was developed by a scientific team of researchers for the AWHONN. More than 30 geographically diverse project sites in California, Colorado, Connecticut, Delaware, Iowa, Kansas, Kentucky, Michigan, Missouri, Nebraska, New Jersey, New York, North Carolina, Ohio, Pennsylvania, Rhode Island, Texas, and Washington D.C. are using this research-based protocol.

Nurse practitioners in a New York hospital are also using research-based protocols to change practice; for example, use of a heparin bolus so that femoral arterial sheaths can be removed sooner, resulting in less time in bed and less discomfort for patients, has become standardized in the cardiac catheterization lab (Wald, 1998). Another interesting example of research use, described by Kilpack, Boehm, Smith, and Mudge (1991), shows how using research-based interventions helped to decrease patient falls.

As a nurse, whatever your position or wherever you work, you need to keep abreast of and evaluate the research reported in the literature of your field of interest. Many practice-based journals provide user-friendly columns that encourage practicing nurses to use research findings. For example, the *American Journal of Nursing* features an ongoing column "Research for Practice," in which the findings from studies on a variety of clinically relevant topics are described and synthesized (Winslow & Jacobson, 1997). Attending research presentations at professional meetings, conferences, or continuing education offerings is one way of learning about current research. You might also consider forming or joining a journal club. Journal clubs have a long history and involve small groups of practitioners or students, or both, meeting on an ongoing basis to discuss and critique the latest literature. Finding research-based evidence about the effectiveness of interventions can be challenging. (See chapter 4 for helpful hints on how to search the literature.) When you find a study that appears to have been soundly done and in which the conclusions seem logical, you will want to try out the findings in your practice. As you do this, you may even find additional areas needing study.

RESEARCH AND NURSING RESEARCH DEFINED

According to *Webster's New World College Dictionary* (Neufeldt, 1997, p. 1141), research is "a careful, systematic, patient study and investigation in some field of knowledge, undertaken to discover or establish facts or principles—to search—go over or look through for the purpose of finding something; to explore; examine for something concealed." Nursing research might discover a concealed treasure!

In the strictest sense, nursing research is concerned with the systematic investigation of nursing practice itself and of the effect of this practice on patient care or on individual, family, or community health. This statement is not meant to imply that research in nursing education or in the administration of nursing service is not vitally important; it is, but it is not strictly nursing research. Rather, it is educational research in nursing, or it is nursing administration research. Albrecht and Herbener's (1992) descriptive study of nurse educators' perceptions and use of nursing educator research findings typifies the former. For an example of the latter, Ballard (1995) describes the need for well-prepared nurse administrators in long-term care. These approaches are commonly included in the general term "nursing research." In fact, all research that is related to nursing, both basic and applied, is considered nursing research by many. Others believe, however, that the term refers to research in nursing practice and in the nursing care needs of patients, that is, clinical research. For an excellent review of factors that encourage and barriers that discourage the use of nursing research findings see the articles by Funk et al. (1991) and Pettengill, Gillies, and Clark (1994). For a frank discussion of nursing research versus research in nursing, you should read Brodie's "Voices in Distant Camps" (1988).

SCIENTIFIC INVESTIGATION AND PROBLEM SOLVING

Scientific inquiry is sometimes compared with problem solving, although the latter is simpler than research is. Perhaps the best way of comparing the two approaches is to compare their uses. Problem solving usually involves finding a solution for an immediate, practical problem. That is, it concerns a problem in client care that cannot wait for research and consists of the following steps used in the nursing process:

1. Assessment—becoming aware of and identifying the particular problem or condition of the client or family that requires care.
2. Diagnosis—analyzing and diagnosing the various aspects of the problem; for example, the need for immediate care, the type of care needed, the need to refer the family for social or financial assistance, and the resources available.
3. Outcome identification—identifying expected outcomes individualized to the client or family and documenting them as measurable goals.
4. Planning—developing a plan of care for the client or family, the problem, and documenting the possible solutions through the use of records, observation, interviews, discussion with other professionals familiar with the client, and review of the pertinent literature.
4. Implementation—analyzing the information collected and using this analysis as a guide to action or nursing intervention in helping the client with the problem.
5. Evaluation—checking with the client or the family, or both, to evaluate the effect of the action taken. If the action fails to solve the problem, start over, looking for alternate solutions (adapted from American Nurses Association, 1997).

The purpose of research is to provide new knowledge by finding valid answers to questions that have been raised or valid solutions to problems that have been identified. Unlike problem solving, the problem selected for research is not related to a particular patient or immediate concern; rather, it is related to the care of patients generally or to a particular group of patients, and the expectation is that the results of the research will benefit many patients.

An investigation that seeks to find solutions to a practical problem, for example, a problem in clinical nursing practice, is called applied research. New knowledge derived from applied research will be useful and can be applied in the field without much delay. Basic research, on the other hand, is not concerned with a here-and-now practical problem; it is concerned with the establishment of new knowledge or facts and the development of fundamental theories that will not always be immediately applicable.

Most of the studies in nursing have been applied research. Both types of research are important and necessary, however, and more nurses should become interested in basic research. As Hinshaw (1989) noted, "Nursing is entering a new era, moving from the stage of establishing structures to support nursing research, and building the cadre of scientists needed to conduct investigations, to the stage of focusing on the identification and study of the phenomena which comprise the body of knowledge needed for practice" (p. 162). Examples of basic research done by nurses are Gunderson and Stoeckle's (1995) study "Endotracheal Suctioning of the Newborn Piglet" and the study by Bond, Heitkemper, and Perigo (1996), in which gastric emptying and gastrointestinal (GI) transit in rats with varying ovarian hormone status were compared to define direct ovarian hormone effects on GI function. These examples of basic research will not produce immediate answers to nursing problems, but the knowledge discovered regarding techniques of endotracheal suctioning might provide basic scientific knowledge on which further research can be based, and the information about the effects of the ovarian hormones on GI function in rats could eventually make a contribution to both physiology and nursing. This knowledge might someday assist health care providers in planning therapies for individuals distressed by irritable bowel syndrome and other dysfunctional bowel conditions.

There is a continuing need for development of biological studies to support biobehavioral research at the NINR (Sigmon, Amende, & Grady, 1996). In 1993, a 10-year plan projected that NINR support for the biological sciences would produce biobehavioral research ready to be tested in clinical trials by the year 2000 (Cowan, Heinrich, Lucas, Sigmon, & Hinshaw, 1993). For an excellent review of the use of physiological variables in nursing research reports published from 1989 to 1993 see Pugh and DeKeyser (1995).

Simply stated, scientific research, whether basic or applied, involves the following steps:

1. Identifying the problem, delineating it clearly, and delimiting it to a manageable research question or hypothesis (see chapter 3).
2. Collecting essential facts pertaining to the problem. This includes reviewing the literature, validating the significance of the problem, and selecting or developing theories to explain the problem and to suggest its solution (see chapters 4 and 10).
3. Asking broad research questions or formulating a prediction of an expected outcome, called a hypothesis (pl., hypotheses) (see chapter 5).
4. Setting up a suitable design or method for the study (see chapter 6).
5. Collecting the essential data (facts) required for answering the

research questions or evaluating the hypothesis (see chapters 7 and 10).
6. Analyzing the data and interpreting the results (see chapters 8, 9, and 10).
7. Communicating the findings of the research (see chapter 11).

Each of these steps may be simple or complex, depending on the nature and complexity of the problem studied. Regardless of complexity, however, research must follow these general steps as carefully as possible and be conducted with complete objectivity and honesty.

The implication, then, is that research may, be done for one or more of several reasons: (1) to study the various aspects of a problem of care; for example, Schroeder (1996) used qualitative methods to explore problems associated with imposed bed rest in women experiencing complicated or high-risk pregnancies; (2) to compare two or more methods of care, for example, the study that compared time required to rewarm, incidence of shivering, and nurses' preference in hypothermic postoperative cardiac surgery patients treated with radiant heat versus forced warm air (Giuffre, Heidenreich, & Pruitt, 1994); (3) to evaluate the use of a specific approach to care, which usually involves comparing the approach used with one group to that used with a control group, such as the randomized trial to assess the effectiveness of early discharge and nurse specialist transitional follow-up care of low birth weight infants described by Brooten and colleagues (1986); or (4) to evaluate a theory of nursing (Fawcett & Downs, 1992).

To summarize, research may seek new facts by (1) exploring, describing, and analyzing a situation or problem; (2) making a critical interpretation of facts already known; or (3) discovering new relationships among facts by means of experimentation. The first type of research commonly involves a descriptive or analytical approach, the second involves a historical or documentary approach, and the third involves an experimental or explanatory approach.

OVERVIEW OF TYPES OF RESEARCH

Research studies are often categorized as being quantitative or qualitative. Quantitative research involves a formal, objective, systematic process that uses numerical data and statistical procedures to describe or assess relationships between and among variables. Quantitative research methods can be classified as descriptive, correlational, quasi-experimental, and experimental (see chapter 6). Qualitative research relies less on numbers and measurements and more on observations and interpersonal communication that provide a holistic view of the subject's experiences without limiting questions or responses. Qualitative approaches, which will be discussed later in this chapter and in chapter 6, are often used when little is known about a phenomenon.

Descriptive Research

Descriptive research explores and describes what is and analyzes the findings in relation to their significance. This approach, which relies on both qualitative and quantitative methods, is appropriate when little is known about a phenomenon. Much of nursing research is descriptive. It is often done for the important purpose of generating hypotheses for future correlational and experimental studies, or it may simply be a way of finding out what the facts are (for example, by means of a survey). In nursing there is great need for research that is conducted for the purpose of developing theories or hypotheses to be tested, since "hunches" about approaches to care frequently occur as a result of carefully made and analyzed observations. Collection of such data is, therefore, an important step that frequently needs to be taken prior to the initiation of scientific experimentation. Many different data collection techniques are used in this type of research, including observations, interviewing, preparing surveys, and case studies (see chapter 7 for methods of data collection). Examples of descriptive research in nursing can be found readily in the literature:

- Byra-Cook, Dracup, and Lazik (1990) examined the differences in correlations between two arm sites and two listening surfaces of the stethoscope on the auscultated (indirect) and invasive (direct) measurement of arterial blood pressure in 50 critical care patients, ages ranging from 18 to 70. Fifty percent of the subjects were female. Findings suggest that systolic determination with the bell is more accurate than the diaphragm is in the antecubital fossa but that the diaphragm appears to be more accurate for the diastolic.
- Using a comparative descriptive design, Lander, Fowler-Kerry, and Hill (1990) studied the differences between genders in experiencing pain. Self-report scales were administered to three groups of subjects: 200 children receiving immunization, 75 postsurgical patients with abdominal wounds, and 78 patients suffering from knee pain. Perceptions of pain did not differ between genders.
- The effect of marital support and support from other adults on the emotional and physical adjustment of 121 husbands of women with breast cancer was examined in a descriptive longitudinal study in which women and their partners completed question-

naires at 7 to 10 days and at 1, 2, 3, 6, and 12 months after surgery. Emotional adjustment could be predicted by satisfaction with the patient's response to interactional and emotional needs and by support from other adults at concurrent times, across contiguous times, and from the 7- to10-day postsurgical period to both the 6-month and 1-year end points. Physical adjustment was predicted by support only at selected times (Hoskins et al., 1996).
- "Breastfeeding Success with Preterm Quadruplets" (Mead, Chuffo, Lawlor-Klean, & Meier, 1992) is an example of a descriptive case study reporting the authors' management of the mother's in-hospital breast-feeding experiences according to research-based guidelines for breast-feeding preterm neonates and infants.

Experimental Research

Whereas the investigator who uses the descriptive method makes observations under natural conditions, an investigator using an experimental or explanatory method manipulates the situation in some way in order to test the hypothesis (or hypotheses) that has been made. A controlled situation is set up; that is, certain factors, or variables, are held constant, an independent or experimental variable is manipulated, and the results are evaluated and compared with the results obtained in the controlled group (see chapter 6 for definitions of these terms). Usually at least one control group and one experimental group are used.

The purposes of experimental studies may be to determine or explain why something happens, to see whether a predicted result occurs when a specific type of care is given, or to evaluate a new program or project. The continuing development of nursing science is in no small part dependent on sound experimental research. Some examples of this type of research in nursing include the following:

- To test the effects of a social support boosting intervention on stress, coping, and social support of caregivers of children with HIV/AIDS, a team of nurse researchers (Hansell et al., 1998) conducted an experimental study in which caregivers (biological parents, extended family members, and foster parents) were randomly assigned to a group receiving a monthly social support boosting intervention (experimental group) or standard care (control group). Levels of stress, coping, and social support were assessed on entry into the study and at 6 months and 1 year. Seronegative caregivers in the experimental group showed significantly increased levels of social support at 6 months as compared with seronegative caregivers in the control group and seropositive caregivers in both groups. There were no significant findings for stress or coping. This study demonstrates the potential benefits of a social support boosting intervention for seronegative caregivers (extended family members and foster parents) of children with HIV/AIDS.

- Miller and Perry (1990) used a two-group pretest and posttest quasi-experimental design to determine how effective a slow deep-breathing technique would be to relieve postoperative pain after CABG surgery. They divided a convenience sample of 29 subjects into an experimental group ($n = 15$) that was taught the relaxation technique on the preoperative evening and performed it postoperatively and a control group ($n = 14$) that did not receive the relaxation training. Analysis of variance (ANOVA) showed no significant decrease of analgesic use but did show significant decreases in the experimental group in blood pressure, heart rate, respiratory rate, and report of pain on a visual descriptor scale. Experimental group subjects were unanimous in evaluating the relaxation technique as simple to do and in stating that they would recommend it to others to decrease postoperative pain.
- Vessey, Carlson, and McGill (1994) investigated the effectiveness of a distraction technique in reducing a child's perceived pain and behavioral distress during an acute pain experience. A sample of 100 children ages 3 through 12 years scheduled for routine blood draws was recruited, and the children were randomly assigned to an experimental or control group. During venipuncture, the control subjects received standard preparation, which consisted of being comforted by physical touch and soft voices; experimental subjects were encouraged to use a kaleidoscope as a distraction technique. Results indicated a significant difference between the groups. The experimental group perceived less pain and demonstrated less behavioral distress than did the control group.

Qualitative Research

The purpose of qualitative research is to explore and illuminate characteristics of human experiences about which little is known or understood in the context in which they occur using rich descriptions provided by the participants (Shurpin & Dumas, 1998). Qualitative research, in contrast to the deductive process of quantitative research, starts from an inductive process (see chapter 1). It is more concerned with description and subjective lived experience rather than with statistical inferences. The investigator formulates a very general research question from clinical experience or observation. The kinds of problems that arise in clinical practice easily lend themselves to a qualitative methodological approach. Shurpin and Dumas (1998, p. 1) note,

> The nature of the interactions which nurses have with patients and their families provide an ideal setting in which nurses can learn more about the human experience and phenomena arising in health care. A qualitative approach is particularly well suited to describe the nurse-patient communication and caring behaviors, which characterize nursing practice.

Qualitative research is an interactive methodology in which the researcher organizes and interprets observations, providing a holistic view of the participant's experiences without limiting questions or responses (Feldman & Hott, 1991). As Munhall (1992) says, "The researcher wishes to understand the meaning an experience has for other human beings and understand the mysteries of the commonplace as well as the unique" (p. 259). In "It Takes Two to Breastfeed: The Baby's Role in Successful Breastfeeding," Lothian (1995) described how she designed a qualitative study to capture the complexities of the experience of breast-feeding as it evolved over time. Her initial research question was, "What is the experience of breast-feeding?" Over time, the focus of the study became, "What influences women to continue to breast-feed?"

There are several approaches used in qualitative research. Phenomenology is a rigorous, critical, systematic investigation of a phenomenon central to the life experience of human beings and about which little has been previously documented (Carpenter, 1995). Shaw (1997) used this approach to describe the lived experience of the death of a peer during adolescence. She interviewed eight women who wished to describe and discuss their experience of the death of an adolescent peer and the impact it had on their subsequent development. From their lived experience emerged a sense of meaning, truth, and reality regarding their perception of this phenomenon. Ethnography is a qualitative approach to research in which the investigator learns about a particular culture or situation by becoming a part of the culture or situation under investigation. Killion (1995) used this approach to study homeless pregnant women in Southern California. The intense social interaction with the women in their own milieu allowed the researcher to witness the homeless experience through the eyes of the women. Grounded theory is another qualitative approach in which data collection and analysis are concurrent and ongoing, with more specific data collected based on the analysis of initial data. Grounded theory uses both an inductive and a deductive approach to theory development.

Olshansky has written extensively on the use and process of grounded theory and employed it in her studies of women's infertility (Olshansky, 1987, 1990, 1996; Woods, Olshansky, & Draye, 1991).

Methods of data collection used in qualitative research usually include participant observation and in-depth interviewing (see chapter 7). In the study mentioned earlier, Lothian (1995) described how participant observation and informal interview provided rich contextual data about the families, their decisions to breast-feed or not, and, subsequently, their experiences of breast-feeding as they actually unfolded over the course of 1 year after the birth of the babies. The case study approach used with a mother who successfully breast-fed quadruplets (Mead et al., 1992) illustrates the use of qualitative research for a nursing problem that is clinically significant (breast-feeding of preterm multiple neonates) but that does not occur with enough frequency for a quantitative or statistical study. Tiller (1993) cites sample size to differentiate between quantitative and qualitative studies. "If the sample size for a quantitative study is small (fewer than 10 subjects), the results may not be conclusive because there were not enough subjects to answer the question. A large sample (more than 500 subjects) may provide different results; however, the study may not be significant. For a qualitative study, a sample size of 8 to 10 is usually appropriate" (p. 13). In the Shaw (1997) study, the sample size was not predetermined but was limited to eight based on the richness and quantity of the data obtained and the extent to which the phenomenon was explored in the interview. The point of data saturation (when information becomes repetitive) decided the number of participants. Sandelowski (1995) provides an excellent reference on "Sample Size in Qualitative Research." She explains that determining adequate sample size in qualitative research is ultimately a matter of judgment and experience in evaluating the quality of the information collected against the use to which it will be put, the particular research method and purposeful sampling strategy employed, and the research product intended.

Rissmiller (1991) provides a very clear comparison between "Qualitative or Quantitative." She comments, "Rather than worry about justifying its use of qualitative approach in research studies, nursing need only feel confident that, if used correctly, such an approach can serve it well" (p. E4). Sandelowski (1997) cautions that despite its growing popularity, qualitative research is often inappropriately used. For example, some researchers attempt to generalize findings from qualitative studies. She explains that "Qualitative research seems warm and fuzzy next to the rigors and demands of statistical work and therefore draws to its ranks persons without the requisite training, talent, and skills. As a result of poor training and misunderstanding, many researchers have legitimated poor scholarship in the name of qualitative research" (1997, p. 127). Mariano (1990), while describing qualitative research as "interactive; context dependent; holistic; flexible, dynamic, and evolving; naturalistic; process oriented; primarily inductive; and descriptive" (p. 354), makes the point that "most nurse researchers, with the possible exception of nurse anthropologists, sociologists, and historians, may have had little exposure to, or experience with, the qualitative method, and academic institutions need to commit time and resources for the development of faculty expertise in this type of inquiry" (p. 359). This is a case of "let the buyer beware" (caveat emptor) for prospective graduate students contemplating qualitative research. (Qualitative methods will be discussed further in chapters 6 and 7.)

Historical Research

Although historical or documentary research has been the type least frequently used by nurse researchers, there appears to be an upswing in historiography. There have been few historiographers in our profession, although histories of nursing were compiled by Nutting and Dock (1907), Dock (1912), Dock and Stewart (1920), Stewart and Austin (1962), and others. According to Christy (1972), historical research follows a specific research methodology and is as concerned with validity and reliability of data as are other types of research. This nurse historian wrote several carefully researched and documented biographical articles on such leaders in nursing as Annie W. Goodrich, M. Adelaide Nutting, and Lillian D. Wald (Christy, 1969a, 1969b, 1969c, 1969d, 1970a, 1970b). Three other examples of carefully documented historical research are Palmer's articles, "Florence Nightingale and the Salisbury Incident" (1976) and "Florence Nightingale and International Origins of Modern Nursing" (1981), and one on the experiences of nurses on Bataan and Corregidor by Kalisch and Kalisch (1976). Austin's (1971) biography of the Woolsey sisters and Woodham-Smith's biography of Florence Nightingale (1951) are examples of carefully documented, book-length works. Stella Goostray's *Memoirs: Half a Century in Nursing* (1969) is a book of one individual's remembrances and thus may not be as well-documented as biographies are. Such writings are most useful in giving impressions of a period in nursing, however. Carnegie's two editions of "The Path We Tread" (1986, 1991) provide sociopolitical and cultural historical background for Black nurses in this country.

In her president's message to the American Association for the History of Nursing (AAHN), Brodie asked, "Does the act of being a nurse historian serve to infuse one's work with a special understanding of the profession's past, or does it compromise one's objectivity? And, does one's need to justify constantly the value of historical scholarship to nursing peers influence either one's objectivity, or limit one's willingness to study all aspects of nursing, even the negative side?" (1991, p. 2). Brodie predicted that future nurse historians will move away from studying advances and achievements to analyzing the sources, problems, and processes of professional growth.

The value of historical research is not merely that it provides a record of the past but that it also contributes to present thought and decision making regarding the future. The old saying that "history repeats itself" is often interpreted to mean that we tend to repeat our failures. Much, however, can be learned from history that will help to explain the present and to broaden our perspective concerning today's problems. According to one author, history's value lies in its ability to help clarify the context in which today's problems exist (Fischer, 1970, pp. 315–316). Furthermore, it contributes to the solution of future problems by adding another dimension to our theoretical knowledge. (For example, what were the conditions under which nursing made significant progress and what were those under which it faltered?) It helps to think historically, to take stock, and to determine new directions. See Anderson's article, "Ethel Fenwick's Legacy to Nursing and Women," for an illustration of the importance of understanding the past and its influence on the future (1981).

The increasing number of doctoral dissertations and articles that are based on historical research and the burgeoning historical societies in nursing reflects a growing interest among nurses in this type of research. There has been a tremendous upsurge in interest in nursing history among historians and other scholars. This interest is reflected in publications such as Melosh's *The Physician's Hand: Work Culture and Conflict in American Nursing* (1982) and in historical documentary films, such as *Sentimental Women Need Not Apply* (Florentine Films, 1988), *Nursing in America—A History of Social Reform* (National League for Nursing, 1990), and *Handmaidens and Battle-Axes* (Silver Films, 1990), which is a history of international nursing.

The AAHN has sponsored annual conferences since 1984. The conference provides a forum for sharing historical research on nursing (American Association for the History of Nursing, 1998). The Center for the Study of The History of Nursing was established in 1985 to encourage and facilitate historical scholarship on health care history and nursing in the United States. The Center continues to create and maintain a resource for such research; to improve the quality of and scope of historical scholarship on nursing; and to disseminate new knowledge on nursing history through education, conferences, publications, and interdisciplinary collaboration (The Chronicle, 1997). In 1997, the governing body of the ICN adopted a resolution supporting national nurses' associations and partner organizations in their efforts to reappraise their national history and tradition of nursing and to promote the awareness of the importance of the history of nursing at the international level and disseminate findings on the history of nursing (ICN, 1997). Lavinia Dock would be proud to see how historical research is now alive and well.

For a further exposition of the methods used in historical research, read the classic works of Christy, "Characteristics of Historical Research and Problems of the Historian" (1972) and "The Methodology of Historical Research: A Brief Introduction" (1975), and Monteiro's "Research into Things Past: Tracking Down One of Miss Nightingale's Correspondents" (1972). In "Historical Research in Nursing: Standards for Research and Evaluation," Hewitt (1997) looked at 11 more recent historical nursing research articles. She describes historical research as a method of inquiry that combines science and literature and suggests that an informed understanding of nursing history provides insights that can contribute effective approaches to current professional issues. In "Historical Methodology for Nursing Research," Lusk (1997) described basic tenets of historical research methodologies. She concluded that historical research is a type of scholarly inquiry and requires attention to methodology. Birnback, Brown, and Hiestand (1993) describe ethical guidelines for the nurse historian. Periodically, journals have devoted entire issues to nursing history (see *Image: Journal of Nursing Scholarship,* 1997; *Nursing Research,* 1987, 1992; *Advances in Nursing Science,* 1985). The entire Fall 1997 issue of *Reflections* was devoted to history by decades, with different nurse historians writing about each decade. For a comprehensive overview of the history of nursing research see D'Antinio's (1997) article, "Toward a History of Research in Nursing." (See chapter 6 for more on methodologies used in historical research.)

Legal Research

Kjervik and King (1990) have suggested that legal research is a method that can be drawn on by nurse researchers to respond to policy questions in the domain of nursing care, for example, "the legal parameters of nursing practice standards, the nature of informed consent in the patient care context, and the elements of nursing employment relationships" (p. 213). The legal research method can enhance nursing's phenomenological approach to studying nursing's problems by understanding human experience from the individual's perspective. Legal research is a way to reach primary legal authority. Conventionally archival in nature, it seeks out written legal authority in case law, legislative acts, and executive arm pronouncements, but it is also qualitative in its inductive and descriptive approach.

A growing number of legal nurse consultant certificate programs have emerged across the country (American Association of Legal Nurse Consultants, 1998). Legal nurse consultants are responsible for reviewing malpractice claims, analyzing the legal impact of medical decisions, conducting criminal and forensic investigations, accompanying attorneys to depositions and much more (Hofstra University, 1997). Many nurses are also attending law school and becoming nurse attorneys. If you are interested in current articles written by respected and experienced nurses and nurse attorneys you are encouraged to see *The Journal of Nursing Law.* This journal, endorsed by The American Association of Nurse Attorneys (TAANA), is a comprehensive guide to key legal issues in the dramatically changing health care field (American Association of Nurse Attorneys, 1998). As the nursing profession produces more nurse attorneys, and legal nurse consultants, legal research will become another important nursing research technique.

ETHICAL ASPECTS OF NURSING RESEARCH

In recent years, considerable concern has been expressed about the protection of the rights of individuals used as subjects of research. Primary factors involved in such protection are (1) informed and voluntary consent on the part of the subject, (2) confidentiality of the data collected, and (3) protection of the individual from harm.

Moral principles have guided human conduct over the centuries in all societies. In our own society, Judeo-Christian ethics or beliefs and values have been the major influence on our standards of human behavior. These values are clearly expressed constitutionally in our belief in the worth and dignity of humans and their right to the pursuit of life, liberty, and happiness.

Organized nursing has expressed its beliefs in its codes of ethics. These have been concerned mainly with ethical conduct in the practice of nursing; recent codes have included ethical considerations with respect to the nurse and research (American Nurses Association, 1968a, 1976, 1985). The 1976 code spoke to the nurse's responsibility to conduct systematic investigations for the purpose of enlarging the body of scientific knowledge basic to nursing and to the patient's rights to privacy, to informed consent, and to be treated with human dignity.

The ANA issued its first ethical guidelines for the nurse in research in 1968 (American Nurses Association, 1968b). Major emphasis was on the protection of human rights: privacy, self-determination, conservation of personal resources, freedom from harm, freedom from intrinsic risk of injury, and informed consent of responsible relatives for minors or incompetent persons.

In 1975, the ANA issued a new statement, entitled *Human Rights Guidelines for Nurses in Clinical and Other Research* (American Nurses Association, 1975). Human rights are discussed under two major aspects: the right to freedom from intrinsic risk of injury and the right to privacy and dignity. These two rights are spelled out in detail and cover all aspects of freedom from harm and the right to privacy, confidentiality, anonymity, and human dignity, as well as freedom from exploitation, especially for those who are members of "vulnerable" populations, such as children, the mentally or emotionally disabled, the physically disabled, institutionalized individuals, and pregnant women. The guidelines also discuss the protection of human rights for nurses in two roles: as investigators and as practitioners who become involved in clinical investigations carried out by practitioners in other fields. In the latter case, protection of human rights extends to the nurses who participate by carrying out investigative practices as well as to the subjects of these practices. This protection holds true no matter who the investigator is, whether physician, nurse, or other researcher.

These guidelines go on to discuss the two major mechanisms by which human rights are protected (American Nurses Association, 1975). First, free and informed consent must characterize the method of obtaining subjects. This consent must be given voluntarily. Subjects, or their legal representatives, must have the freedom to participate or not and to withdraw from an investigation whenever they so desire. Second, there is the need for a review committee within the institution representing the various occupational groups to review all research proposals. Further, the guidelines propose that the ANA actively support the appointment of competent nurses as members of these review committees. Today, most institutions with research programs involving human subjects have such committees and institutional review boards to review and approve all research proposals. Their review is concerned not only with the significance of the study and the soundness of the research design but also with the evidence that the subjects' rights will be protected. For a comprehensive discussion of institutional review boards or committees, see Nokes (1989) and the U.S. Department of Health and Human Services publication, *Protecting Human Research Subjects: Institutional Review Board Guidebook* (1993).

Obtaining informed consent from human subjects must be given careful consideration in order to conduct ethical research (Berry, Dodd, Hinds, & Ferrell, 1996; Davis, 1989; Rempusheski, 1991; Trudeau, 1993). If you plan a research project in which human beings are the subjects, you need to consider the kind of explanation that will be required for the subject to understand the nature of the project. In the experimental study of caregivers of children with HIV/AIDS, described earlier in this chapter, special care was required in obtaining informed consent due to confidentiality issues with this vulnerable population.

In some situations, it may not be necessary to give a complete description of the project and its purposes, if doing so would ruin your chances of obtaining the data you need. You do not want to tip your hand and influence the outcome of the study. For example, in the Rentschler (1991) study of correlates of successful breast-feeding, volunteers were recruited through prepared childbirth classes. Participants were given verbal explanation of the purpose of the study and the procedure for collecting data. Mothers were told that the researcher wanted to learn about factors related to infant feeding. The participating mothers were not told that the researcher was specifically interested in factors related to "successful" breast-feeding, that is, breast-feeding for at least 6 weeks. This knowledge might have colored their responses and directly or indirectly influenced the length of successful breast-feeding. When the full nature of the research purpose cannot be disclosed to the subjects, as in this example, the review and approval by an institutional review board or committee becomes particularly important.

The Nurse's Responsibility

All nurses involved in research in any way, as a researcher, as a participant in someone else's research, or even as a subject of research, must be informed about the rights of human subjects. There are legal as well as ethical responsibilities involved. It is recommended that you read and discuss the ANA guidelines and two classic articles: "Ethics of Nursing Research: Profile, Principles, Perspective" by Sister Bernadette Armiger (1977) and "Legal Concerns of Nursing Research" by Helen Creighton (1977). Other references of special interest are "Ethical Issues in Conducting Clinical Nursing Research" (Collins, 1993); "Clinical Research: Considerations for Prospective Participants" (Hutchins & Eckes, 1996); and "Ethical Guidelines in the Conduct, Dissemination & Implementation of Nursing Research" (Silva, 1995). Eisch, Colling, Ouslander, Hadley, and Campbell (1991) discuss the challenges and difficulty of accessing patients in nursing home settings, and Akers and Bell (1994) ask whether children should be used as research subjects. Children and the consent process are also addressed by Broome and Stieglitz (1992). McGrath (1995) emphatically presents a case for saying no in a discussion of ethical issues arising from informed consent to chemotherapy. Dieckmann and Smith (1989) provide very good "how to" strategies for gaining institutional access, recruiting subjects, obtaining informed consent, and using advertising and incentives for participants. Incentives are often aimed at reducing attrition. For example, in the study on caregivers of children with HIV/AIDS funded by NINR, the researcher built the cost of providing incentives into the budget of the grant (Hansell et al., 1998). Participants received $50.00 after they completed the questionnaires at 6 months and 1 year as a way of thanking them for participating. Many researchers provide a stamped return envelope and promise to share a summary of results with those who participate. The reason token financial incentives have been found so effective in research may lie not in their monetary value but rather in the fact that they are a symbol of trust. They represent the researcher's trust that the respondent will accept an offer made in good faith. Second, incentives may stimulate the belief on the part of the participant that future promises (e.g., a copy of results or putting the results to good use) will be carried out (Dillmann, 1978).

SUMMARY

In this chapter we have discussed why research is done, the responsibility that you as a nurse have for participating in research, and the ethical considerations involved in all research. We have also introduced some of the types of research and given examples of each. It should not be inferred that any one type of research is better than another; all demand the best efforts of the investigator. What is important is that the type of research selected is the right one for the problem to be studied and the purpose of the study.

Research is serious business. It should not be entered into lightly, but neither should it be feared. It can be the most exciting, demanding, addicting, and rewarding of experiences for the amateur as well as the pro. As the old commercial says, "Try it; you'll like it!"; or, as the more recent Nike ad says, "Just do it!"

REFERENCES

Advances in Nursing Science. (1985). *7*(2), 1–83.

Akers, J., & Bell, S. (1994). Should children be used as research subjects? *Nursing Forum, 29*(3), 28–33.

Albrecht, S. A., & Herbener, D. J. (1992, June 17). *Summary of results: Nurse educators' perceptions and use of nursing education research findings.* University of Pittsburgh, School of Nursing: personal correspondence.

American Association for the History of Nursing (AAHN). (1998, January 14). [On-line]. Available: http://users.aol.com/NsgHistory/AAHN.html.

American Association of Legal Nurse Consultants. (1998, February 6). [On-line]. Available: http://www.aalnc.org/index.html.

American Association of Nurse Attorneys. (1998, February 6). [On-line]. Available: http://www.aalnc.org/index.htm.

American Nurses Association. (1968a). *Code for nurses with interpretative statements.* New York: Author.

American Nurses Association. (1968b). *The nurse in research: ANA guidelines on ethical values.* New York: Author.

American Nurses Association. (1975). *Human rights guidelines for nurses in clinical and other research.* Kansas City, MO: Author.

American Nurses Association. (1976). *Code for nurses with interpretative statements.* Kansas City, MO: Author.

American Nurses Association. (1997). *Standards of clinical nursing practice.* Washington, DC: Author.

Anderson, N. D. (1981). Ethel Fenwick's legacy to nursing and women. *Image, 13,* 32–33.

Armiger, B. (1977). Ethics of nursing research: Profile, principles, perspective. *Nursing Research, 26,* 330–336.

Association for Women's Health, Obstetric and Neonatal Nurses (AWHONN). (1998). *Preliminary program.* AWHONN, Association of Women's Health, Obstetric and Neonatal Nurses, 1998 Convention: Forging New Frontiers, San Antonio, Texas.

Austin, A. L. (1971). *The Woolsey sisters of New York, 1860–1900.* Philadelphia: American Philosophical Society.

Ballard, T. (1995). The need for well-prepared nurse administrators in long-term care. *Image, 27*(2), 153–154.

Beck, C. T. (1994). Replication strategies for nursing research. *Image, 26*(3), 191–194.

Berry, D., Dodd, M., Hinds, P., & Ferrell, B. (1996). Ethical issues. Informed consent: process and clinical issues. *Oncology Nursing Forum, 23,* 507–512.

Birnbach, N., Brown, J., & Hiestand, W. (1993). Ethical guidelines for the nurse historian. Standards of professional conduct for historical inquiry in nursing. *American Association for the History of Nursing Bulletin, 38,* 4–5.

Bond, E., Heitkemper, M., & Perigo, R. (1996). Gastric emptying and gastric-intestinal transit in rats with varying ovarian hormone status. *Nursing Research, 45*(4), 218–224.

Bookbinder, M. (1992a). *Nurse linkage agents' efforts to facilitate the use of a research-based innovation.* Unpublished doctoral dissertation, New York University, New York.

Bookbinder, M. (1992b). Research: What's in it for you? *Nursing Spectrum: Greater New York/Tri-State Edition, 4*(2), 8.

Bookbinder, M. (1992c). Searching for solutions. *Nursing Spectrum: Greater New York/Tri-State Edition, 4*(10).

Brodie, B. (1988). Voices in distant camps: The gap between nursing research and nursing practice. *Journal of Professional Nursing, 4,* 320–328.

Brodie, B. (1991). President's message: Musings of a nurse historian on being a nurse historian. *AAHN Bulletin, 32,* 2.

Broome, M., & Stieglitz, K. (1992). The consent process and children. *Research in Nursing and Health, 15*(2), 147–152.

Brooten, D., Kumar, S., Brown, L., Butts, P., Finkler, S. A., Bakewell-Sachs, S., Gibbons, A., & Delivoria-Papadopoulos, M. (1986). A randomized trial of early hospital discharge and home follow-up of very low-birth weight infants. *New England Journal of Medicine, 315,* 934–939.

Budin, W. (1998). Psychosocial adjustment to breast cancer in unmarried women. *Research in Nursing and Health, 21,* 155–166.

Byra-Cook, C., Dracup, K., & Lazik, A. (1990). Direct and indirect blood pressure in critical care patients. *Nursing Research, 39,* 285–288.

Campbell, J., Poland, M., Waller, J., & Ager, J. (1992). Correlates of battering during pregnancy. *Research in Nursing and Health, 15*(3), 219–226.

Carnegie, E. (1986). *The path we tread: Blacks in nursing 1854–1984.* Philadelphia: Lippincott.

Carnegie, E. (1991). *The path we tread* (2nd ed.). New York: National League for Nursing.

Carpenter, D. (1995). Phenomenological research approach. In F. Steubert, & D. R. Carpenter (Eds.), *Qualitative research in nursing—advancing the humanistic imperative* (pp. 29–49). Philadelphia: J. B. Lippincott.

Center for the study of the history of nursing: University of Pennsylvania School of Nursing. (1997). *Chronicle, 10*(1), 2.

Christy, T. E. (1969a). Portrait of a leader: Isabel Hampton Robb. *Nursing Outlook, 17,* 26–29.

Christy, T. E. (1969b). Portrait of a leader: Isabel Maitland Stewart. *Nursing Outlook, 17,* 44–48.

Christy, T. E. (1969c). Portrait of a leader: Lavinia Lloyd Dock. *Nursing Outlook, 17,* 72–75.

Christy, T. E. (1969d). Portrait of a leader: M. Adelaide Nutting. *Nursing Outlook, 17,* 202–204.

Christy, T. E. (1970a). Portrait of a leader: Annie Warburton Goodrich. *Nursing Outlook, 18,* 46–50.

Christy, T. E. (1970b). Portrait of a leader: Lillian D. Wald. *Nursing Outlook, 18,* 50–54.

Christy, T. E. (1972). *Characteristics of historical research and problems of the historian.* Proceedings of the American Nurses' Association Eighth Nursing Research Conference (pp. 227–228).

Christy, T. E. (1975). The methodology of historical research: A brief introduction. *Nursing Research, 24,* 189–192.

Collins, B. (1993). Ethical issues in conducting clinical nursing research. *AWHONN's Clinical Issues in Perinatal and Women's Health Nursing, 4,* 620–633.

Cowan, M., Heinrich, J., Lucas, M., Sigmon, H., & Hinshaw, A. S. (1993). Integration of biological and nursing sciences: A ten-year plan to enhance research and training. *Research in Nursing and Health, 16,* 323.

Creighton, H. (1977). Legal concerns of nursing research. *Nursing Research, 26,* 337–341.

D'Antinio, P. (1997). Toward a history of research in nursing. *Nursing Research, 46*(2) 105–110.

Davis, A. (1989). Informed consent process in research protocols: Dilemmas for clinical nurses. *Western Journal of Nursing Research, 11,* 448–457.

Dieckmann, J., & Smith, J. (1989). Strategies for assessment and recruitment of subjects for nursing research. *Western Journal of Nursing Research, 11,* 418–430.

Dillman, D. (1978). *Mail and telephone surveys: The total design method.* New York: John Wiley & Sons.

Dock, L. L. (1912). *A history of nursing* (Vols. 3 and 4). New York: Putnam.

Dock, L. L., & Stewart, I. M. (1920). *A short history of nursing.* New York: Putnam.

Eastern Nursing Research Society (ENRS). (1998). *ENRS membership directory.* Durham, NH: University of New Hampshire Press.

Eisch, J. S., Colling, J., Ouslander, J., Hadley, B. J., & Campbell, E. (1991). Issues in implementing clinical research in nursing settings. *Journal of the New York State Nurses Association, 22,* 18–21.

Elkind, E. (1998). AWHONN researchers develop new nursing protocol. *New Jersey News: AWHONN, 10*(1) 2.

Fahs, P., & Kinney, M. (1991). The abdomen, thigh, and arm as sites for subcutaneous sodium heparin injections. *Nursing Research, 40*(4), 204–207.

Fawcett, J., & Downs, F. (1992). *The relationship of theory and research.* Philadelphia: F. A. Davis.

Feldman, H., Penny, N., Harter, J., Hott, J. R., & Jacobson, L. (1993). Bridging the nursing research-practice gap; through research utilization. *Journal of the New York State Nurses Association, 24*(3), 4–10.

Feldman, H. R., & Hott, J. R. (1991). Light up your practice with nursing research. *Journal of the New York State Nurses Association, 22,* 8–11.

Fischer, D. H. (1970). *Historians' fallacies: Toward a logic of historical thought.* New York: Harper & Row.

Florentine Films. (1988). *Sentimental women need not apply: A history of the American nurse.* [Film]. (Available from Direct Cinema Ltd. Box 10003, Santa Monica, CA 90410. 1-800-525-0000.)

Forman, H. (1997, October). Facets—diamonds or both. *Nursing Spectrum: Greater New York/Tri-State Edition, 20,* 3.

Funk, S., Champagne, M., Wiese, R., & Tornquist, E. (1991). Barriers to using research findings in practice: The clinicians perspective. *Applied Nursing Research, 4,* 90–95.

Goostray, S. (1969). *Memoirs: Half a century in nursing.* Boston: Nursing Archive, Mugar Memorial Library, Boston University.

Giuffre, M., Heidenreich, T., & Pruitt, L. (1994). Rewarming cardiac surgery patients: Radiant heat versus forced warm air. *Nursing Research, 43*(3), 174–178.

Gunderson, L., & Stoeckle, M. (1995). Endotracheal suctioning of the newborn piglet. *Western Journal of Nursing Research, 17,* 20–31.

Hansell, P., Hughes, C., Caliandro, G., Russo, P., Budin, W., Hartman, B., & Hernandez, O. (1998). The effects of a social support boosting intervention on stress, coping, and social support in caregivers of children with HIV/AIDS. *Nursing Research, 47*(2), 79–86.

Henry, B. (Ed.). (1997). Diamond Anniversary Commemorative Edition. *Image: Journal of Nursing Scholarship, 29* (1,2,3,4).

Hewitt, L. (1997). Historical research in nursing: Standards for research and evaluation. *Journal of the New York State Nurses Association, 28*(3), 16–19.

Hinshaw, A. S. (1989). Nursing science: The challenge to develop knowledge. *Nursing Science Quarterly, 2,* 162–171.

Hofstra University. (1997). *Legal nurse consultant certificate program: A new option in the field of law for nurses.* Hempstead, NY: Hofstra University, University College for Continuing Education.

Hoskins, C., Baker, S., Budin, W., Ekstrom, D., Maislin, G., Sherman, D., Steelman-Bohlander, J., Bookbinder, M., & Knauer, C. (1996). Adjustment among husbands of women with breast cancer. *Journal of Psychosocial Oncology, 14*(1), 41–69.

Hoskins, C., Baker, S., Sherman, D., Bohlander, J., Bookbinder, M., Budin, W., Ekstrom, D., Knauer, C., & Maislin, G. (1996). Social support and patterns of adjustment to breast cancer. *Scholarly Inquiry for Nursing Practice: An International Journal, 10*(2), 99–123.

Hutchins, S., & Eckes, R. (1996). Clinical research: Considerations for prospective participants. *Nursing Clinics of North America, 31*(1), 125–135.

International Council of Nurses (ICN). (1997). Resolution adopted by the International Council of Nurse's Governing Body. *Canadian Nurse, 93,* 29.

Kalisch, P., & Kalisch, B. J. (1976). Nurses under fire: The World War II experiences of nurses on Bataan and Corregidor. *Nursing Research, 25,* 409–429.

Killion, C. (1995). Special health needs of homeless pregnant women. *Advances in Nursing Science, 18*(2), 44–56.

Kilpack, B., Boehm, J., Smith, N., & Mudge, B. (1991). Using research based interventions to decrease patient falls. *Applied Research, 4,* 50–56.

Kjervik, D. K., & King, F. E. (1990). The legal research method: An approach to enhance nursing science. *Journal of Professional Nursing, 6,* 213–220.

Kramer, B. (1998). You provide the question, we'll get the answer. *Nursing Spectrum: The New York Metro Edition, 10*(4), 7.

Lander, J., Fowler-Kerry, S., & Hill, A. (1990). Comparison of pain perceptions among males and females. *Canadian Journal of Nursing Research, 22,* 39–49.

Lothian, J. (1995). It takes two to breastfeed: The baby's role in successful breastfeeding. *Journal of Nurse-Midwifery, 40*(4), 328–334.

Lusk, B. (1997). Historical methodology for nursing research. *Image: Journal of Nursing Scholarship, 29*(4), 355–359.

Marks, D. (1996). Workplace issues: Nearly 10 percent of nurses suffer from latex allergy. *American Nurse, 28*(7), 7.

Martin, P. (1995). More replication studies needed. *Applied Nursing Research, 8*(2), 102–103.

Mariano, C. (1990). Qualitative research. *Nursing and Health Care, 11,* 354–359.

McGrath, P. (1995). It's ok to say no! A discussion of ethical issues arising from informed consent to chemotherapy. *Cancer Nursing, 18*(2), 97–103.

Mead, L. J., Chuffo, R., Lawlor-Klean, P., & Meier, P. P. (1992). Breastfeeding success in preterm quadruplets. *Journal of Obstetrical, Gynecological and Neonatal Nursing, 21,* 221–227.

Melosh, B. (1982). *Physician's hand: Work, culture and conflict in American nursing.* Philadelphia: Temple University Press.

Miller, K. M., & Perry, P. A. (1990). Relaxation technique and postoperational pain in patients undergoing cardiac surgery. *Heart & Lung, 19,* 136–146.

Monteiro, L. (1972). Research into things past: Tracking down one of Miss Nightingale's correspondents. *Nursing Research, 22,* 526–529.

Munhall, P. L. (1992). Holding the Mississippi River in place and other implications for qualitative research. *Nursing Outlook, 40*(6), 257–262.

National Institute of Child Health and Human Development (NICHD). (1997). Electronic Fetal Heart Rate Monitoring: Research Guidelines for Interpretation. The National Institute of Child Health and Human Development research Planning Workshop. *Journal of Obstetric, Gynecologic and Neonatal Nursing, 26,* 635–664.

National League for Nursing. (1990). *Nursing in America—history of social reform.* New York: Author.

Neufeldt, V. (Ed.). (1997). *Webster's New World College Dictionary* (3rd ed.). New York: Macmillan.

New York State Nurses Association (NYSNA). (1998). *Report.* The official newsletter of the New York State Nurses Association. 10.

Nokes, K., (1989). Exploring the institutional review board process. *Journal of the New York State Nurses Association, 20*(3), 7–10.

Nursing history. (1985, January). *Advances in Nursing Science, 7*(2), 1–85.

Nursing Research. (1987). *36,* 1–71.

Nursing Research. (1992). *41,* 1–63.

Nutting, M. A., & Dock, L. L. (1907). *A history of nursing* (Vols. 1 and 2). New York: Putnam.

Olshansky, E. (1987). Infertility and career identities. *Health Care for Women International, 8,* 185–196.

Olshansky, E. (1990). Psychosocial implications of pregnancy after infertility. *Journal of Obstetric, Gynecologic and Neonatal Nursing, 1*(3), 342–347.

Olshansky, E. (1996). Theoretical issues in building a grounded theory: Application of an example of a program of research on infertility. *Qualitative Health Research, 6*(3), 394–405.

Palmer, I. S. (1976). Florence Nightingale and the Salisbury incident. *Nursing Research, 25,* 370–377.

Palmer, I. S. (1981). Florence Nightingale and the international origins of modern nursing. *Image, 13,* 28–31.

Pettengill, M., Gillies, D., & Clark, C. (1994). Factors encouraging and discouraging the use of nursing research findings. *Image, 26,* 143–147.

Pugh, L., & DeKeyser, F. (1995). Use of physiologic variables in nursing research. *Image, 27* (4), 273–276.

Reflections. (1997). *23*(3), 3–62.

Rempusheski, V. F. (1989). Building a team of nurse researchers in the clinical setting. *Nursing Scan in Research, 2,* 1.

Rempusheski, V. F. (1991). Elements, perceptions and issues of informed consent. *Applied Nursing Research, 4,* 201–204.

Rentschler, D. (1991). Correlates of successful breastfeeding. *Nursing Research, 23,* 151–154.

Rice, V., & Johnson, J. (1984). Preadmission self-instruction booklets, postadmission exercise performance, and teaching time. *Nursing Research, 33,* 147–151.

Rice, V., Mullin, M., & Jarosz, P. (1992). Preadmission self-instruction effects on postadmission and postoperative indicators in CABG patients: Partial replication and extension. *Research in Nursing and Health, 15*(4), 253–259.

Rissmiller, A. N. (1991). Qualitative or quantitative. (Application for clinical practice.) *Nursing Scan in Research, 4,* 1–4.

Sandelowski, M. (1995). Sample size in qualitative research. *Research in Nursing and Health, 18*(2), 179–183.

Sandelowski, M. (1997). To be of use: Enhancing the utility of qualitative research. *Nursing Outlook, 45,* 125–132.

Saver, C. (1998, January 26). Interdisciplinary Teams in Action. *Nursing Spectrum: Greater New York/Tri-State Edition, 10A*(2), 6–7.

Schepp, K. G. (1991). Factors influencing the coping efforts of mothers of hospitalized children. *Nursing Research, 40,* 42–46.

Schroeder, C. (1996). Women's experience of bed rest in high-risk pregnancy. *Image, 28*(3), 253–258.

Shaw, H. (1997). *Beyond grief: The extended impact of the death of a peer during adolescence among adult women. A phenomenological inquiry.* Unpublished doctoral dissertation. Adelphi University, Garden City, NY.

Shurpin, K., & Dumas, M.A. (1998). Evaluating expert practice in nursing. Contexts: A forum for the Medical Humanities. *The Institute for Medicine in Contemporary Society, 6*(2), 1–2.

Sigmon, H., Amende, L., & Grady, P. (1996). Development of biological studies to support biobehavioral research at the National Institute of Nursing Research, *Image, 28*(2), 88.

Silva, M. (1995). *Ethical guidelines in the conduct, dissemination & implementation of nursing research.* Washington, DC: American Nurses Association.

Silver Films. (1990). *Handmaidens and battleaxes.* [Film]. (Available from Direct Cinema Ltd., Box 10003, Santa Monica, CA 90410. 1-800-525-0000)

Society of Rogerian Scholars. (1998). *Membership directory.* New York: Author. (Available from P.O. Box 1195, Canal Street Station, NY, NY 10013-0867)

Stewart, I. M., & Austin, A. L. (1962). *A history of nursing.* New York: Putnam.

Tiller, C. (1993). Nurse advises how to read research. *AWHONN Voice, 1* (3), 13.

Trudeau, M. (1993). Informed consent: The patient's right to decide. *Journal of Psychosocial Nursing and Mental Health Services, 31*(6), 9–12, 30–32.

U.S. Department of Health and Human Services. (1990). *Seventh report to the President and Congress on the status of health personnel in the United States.* Washington, D.C.: Author.

U.S. Department of Health and Human Services (1993). *Protecting human research subjects: Institutional review board guidebook.* Washington, DC: Author.

Vessey, J., Carlson, K., & McGill, J. (1994). Use of distraction with children during an acute pain experience. *Nursing Research, 43*(6), 369–372.

Wald, A. (1998). New allies for cardiothoracic patients: Nurse practitioners. *Nursing Spectrum: Greater New York Metro Edition, 10*(3), 4–5.

Wilson, H. S. (1991). Identifying problems for clinical research to create a nursing tapestry. *Nursing Outlook, 39,* 280–282.
Winslow, E., & Jacobson, A. (1997). Research for Practice. *American Journal of Nursing, 97*(12), 21.
Woodham-Smith, C. (1951). *Florence Nightingale.* New York: McGraw-Hill.
Woods, N. F., Olshansky, E., & Draye, M. (1991). Infertility: Women's experiences. *Health Care for Women International, 12*(2), 179–190.

PART II

The Research Process

3

Selecting a Problem

As we have found in the two preceding chapters, the purpose of research is to discover unknown facts, explanations, interpretations, and relationships among facts. We have also learned that research may be either basic or applied, descriptive, experimental, qualitative, or historical. From now on, we shall focus on research in clinical nursing, that is, on studies of nursing practice or of the effect of nursing practice on patient care or on individual, family, or community health situations. Our purpose will be to find out how we can systematically discover facts or identify relationships among facts that will help us solve problems in nursing.

The problems investigated in nursing may be relatively simple ones, or they may be so broad and complex as to involve large groups of nurses or patients and thus require a team approach. An example of a simple problem might be the one described by Bookbinder (1992), in which nurses searched and read the literature to see how elevating patients' upper bodies 30 degrees affected their PAP readings when in the PACU. Another example of a simple problem was the observation that alterations in sleep patterns are common after CABG surgery. Although some descriptive data on sleep patterns during hospitalization are available, there have been few attempts at objective measurement of sleep over the course of recovery. This prompted a group of nurse researchers to design a study with the purpose to measure sleep patterns over a 6-month time period after CABG surgery using a wrist-worn actigraph and the Sleep-Rest subscale of the Sickness Impact Profile (Redeker, Mason, Wykpisz, & Glica, 1996). An example of a more complex problem is addressed in a series of randomized clinical trials of early discharge with nurse specialist transitional follow-up care as described by Brooten and colleagues (Brooten, Knapp, et al., 1996; Brooten, Naylor, et al., 1996; Brooten et al., 1995). Testing this model of advanced practice nurse transitional care on a wide variety of patient outcomes and health care costs became the framework for a series of studies using various patient populations including very low birth weight infants; women with cesarean birth, high-risk pregnancies, or hysterectomy; and elders with cardiac medical and surgical diagnoses. Findings consistently demonstrated the effectiveness of the advanced practice nurse transitional care in terms of patient outcomes and cost savings. These examples demonstrate a collaborative team approach in which nurses identified the problem and carried out the study. Imagine the excitement of designing your own research, reporting the results, and basing your own nursing care on the findings! This is a success story for nursing practice and, most of all, a positive change for the patients.

FINDING A PROBLEM

How does one go about choosing a problem to study? Some of the best research questions come not from those individuals whose main focus is research but rather from the clinician who is working with people in some aspect of their health care (Humenick, 1994). You may already have in mind a suitable question about some aspect of patient care that has grown out of your daily work or your background of experiences. For instance, you may have been questioning, as Schepp (1991) did, whether nurses' approaches to mothers might have an effect on the relief of their anxiety and might improve coping. You may question sleep patterns in women after coronary artery bypass surgery as Redeker et al. (1996) did. On the other hand, you may not have any questions or hunches about ways of improving care but may be interested in doing some research. In that case, you might go to the literature and read some of the studies reported in the various nursing journals, such as Feldman and Hott's (1991) report on research by nurses. This will give you a picture of the many kinds of problems other nurses have observed, and such an excursion may stimulate your imagination. You may discover that you have several questions of your own that fall into the "What is?" or "Why is such and such happening?" category. It is good to be curious, critical, and skeptical and to ask questions. Remember, there are no stupid questions! This is the beginning of the intellectual curiosity that is so essential to problem identification. Don't worry about stating your question in proper research format . . . just capture the essence.

The nursing process itself is analogous to research activity. In chapter 2 the parallels between assessment, planning, implementation, and evaluation and the problem-solving approach used in research were presented. Using the steps of the nursing process, you may identify important problems areas or raise questions appropriate for research.

Of course, the literature is also full of suggestions for study. Many investigations raise as many questions as they answer, if not more. You might even decide to replicate a reported study in order to substantiate, or perhaps refute, its findings or to determine whether the findings are the same when settings or subjects are different (see Beck, 1994).

Review articles are also often an excellent source of suggestions for study. These are articles that review the research done in a particular area and discuss the research that still needs to be done. For example, in an article reviewing research on women and HIV infection, Smeltzer and Whipple (1991) present the state of the science pertaining to what is known about HIV infection and AIDS in women, alerting nurses to these special issues so that the information can be used in education, practice, and research.

Since 1993, *The Online Journal of Knowledge Synthesis for Nursing* has provided comprehensive full-text, critical reviews of research pertinent to clinical practice problems (Sigma Theta Tau International, 1998). By making available timely, synthesized knowledge to guide nursing practice and research, the journal helps the nursing community stay abreast of the vast amount of information published in nursing journals and other published nursing research. Topics covered in past issues included assessment of postpartum depression, coma stimulation, feeding tube placement, agitation in older persons with dementia, maternal role attainment in adolescents, and factors affecting functional status in chronic obstructive pulmonary disease (COPD) (Sigma Theta Tau International, 1998).

In her survey, Lindeman (1975) found that among the top 10% of research priorities under patient welfare at that time were nursing care related to stress reduction, pain alleviation, improving the quality of life for the institutionalized aged, and education of patients. This type of survey report is also a good source of research ideas. Many of the specialty organizations, such as AWHONN, AACN, ONS, and NINR, have identified research priorities. Priorities for funding identified by the NINR for 1995 through 1999 include research into community-based nursing models, AIDS interventions, reducing the effects of cognitive impairments and chronic illnesses, and behavioral factors influencing the immune system (National Institute of Nursing Research, 1993).

A good review of the literature in your particular area of interest not only is an excellent source of problems but also will serve to enrich your background and help you to relate your interests to those of others in the same field. This is not the same kind of literature review you will do after selecting your research problem. You need to have as much understanding of the general area as you can get before deciding on a particular problem. Perhaps you have specialized in the area of your subject and do not need this review, but even if you are familiar with the literature, a review will refresh your knowledge of the area. The *Annual Review of Nursing Research* (Werley, Fitzpatrick, Stevenson, & Norbeck, 1983–present) is helpful in this regard. This landmark series, now in its second decade of publication, draws together and critically reviews all the existing research in specific areas of nursing practice, nursing care delivery, nursing education, and the profession of nursing.

Suppose the question you are interested in relates to the use of computerized instruction in teaching diabetic patients. You would need to be thoroughly familiar not only with the subject of diabetes and the care of diabetic patients but also with the subject of health teaching methods, including computerized instruction. If you had not already acquired this familiarity, it would be the time to do so.

Sometimes you may find inspiration and support for your ideas in a research interest group. Beckstrand and McBride (1990) present a "how to" approach that explains how busy academic and clinical nurses can pool knowledge and conduct significant research. A research interest group also enables experienced and inexperienced nurses to work together and accomplish what they might not have alone. It's collegial and rewarding; graduate students finding this kind of research training invaluable. For a concise, "no frills" description of how to go about defining and clarifying a research problem, read Rempusheski (1990) or see Kahn (1994).

DELIMITING THE PROBLEM

Some problems, of course, may not be researchable. They may be so global that they do not lend themselves to study. A question such as "How can I improve the self-care of diabetic patients?" would be much too broad, although it could well be the first question you ask. "What is the most effective method of teaching diabetic patients how to take their own insulin?" would also be rather indefinite, although again, you might start with this question. (Time for teaching is often difficult to find in a busy clinic, and you want to find the most successful way of teaching patients.) A much more specific question would be, "Can diabetic patients learn to care for themselves and to take their own insulin as effectively through the use of individual computerized instruction as by means of group instruction?" This question could be studied by making a systematic comparison of the two teaching methods.

The next step in determining whether a problem is feasible for research, or at least whether you would be able to study it, is to determine whether the appropriate patients and the resources needed to do the study are available to you. For example, if you are teaching diabetic patients, it might be relatively easy for you to plan a comparative study of the two methods of teaching suggested earlier if resources for making use of the two methods are available. You may have been using the group method of teaching, but at a conference you heard about a computerized program of instruction that would appear to offer a more effective method. You want to try it. Are you able to access the computer program? Are computers available for your use? If not, would it be possible to acquire this equipment? Is cost a factor? Is the computerized program of instruction "user friendly" for those with little computer experience?

The answers to these questions would help you decide on the practicality of the problem for study, but you would also need to know whether methods of comparing the results are available. You would certainly check the literature for appropriate references, such as Brown's "Quality of Reporting in Diabetes Patient Research, 1954–1986" (1990) and her previous "Effects of Educational Interventions in Diabetes Care: A Meta-Analysis of Findings" (1988). You might decide to pretest and posttest your patients in some way and to develop the tests yourself, perhaps with the help of experts. Also, expert opinion might be available for helping you develop a rating scale for evaluating such variables as skin condition, number of complications, handling of injections, and urine testing, to mention a few. You probably would also want to find out about additional ways of rating the effectiveness or outcomes of the two teaching methods.

You may think that we have made much ado about selecting a problem for study. This is one of the most important steps in the whole research process, however; it determines to a large extent the nature and quality of your research. It is often said that once we know what the problem is, we are well on our way to solving it. Problem identification is not always easy (Kahn, 1994). The habit of systematic observation plus intellectual curiosity and a questioning attitude will help, however. A further help is familiarity with the literature, which will provide suggestions for problems that need to be studied (Brown, 1990).

ESTABLISHING THE SIGNIFICANCE OF THE PROBLEM

An important factor in the selection of a problem for study is whether it is an important or significant problem. Is there a real need to find an answer to it? As you review the literature, particularly the research literature, you will see that in most reports the introductory material provides a rationale for the study; that is, it explains the reason the investigator considered the study important. On the face of it, the suggested study of the use of computerized instruction would appear to be of importance because improved learning by diabetic patients should result in better self-care and fewer complications. If several scientific investigations of this problem, using computerized instruction to advantage, have already been reported in the literature, however, you might question the need for doing another study. Nevertheless, the study would be in order if some new element has been added to the instruction method since the previous studies were made or if your evaluation of the studies suggests a need for substantiating the findings.

STATING THE PURPOSE

Once you have identified the problem, you can come up with a clear statement of your purpose in studying it. This will give direction and focus to the study. For example, the purpose of the study we suggested would be to compare the effectiveness of two methods of teaching diabetic patients self-care: group instruction and computerized instruction. The purpose of a study by Engebretson (1996) was to compare concepts of health and healing used by nurses and alternative healers. In another study, the purpose was to "determine the relationships among primary treatment alternative, symptom distress, social support, and psychosocial adjustment to breast cancer in unmarried women" (Budin, 1998). One may argue that the purpose of all three of these studies would be to improve the care of certain patients. This is the ultimate purpose of all nursing research and an indication of the usefulness of the particular study. Although some researchers do include the ultimate reason for the study (to plan better care for these patients, for example), this is not necessarily part of the specific statement of purpose.

The rationale for a study often includes not only the statement of the problem but also the significance and usefulness of the study. The rationale should clearly tie in with and culminate in the statement of the purpose of the research. In the suggested study of methods of teaching the diabetic patient, for example, the importance of teaching these patients effectively would have to be established. Next would come the determination of the need for a solution of the question about the effectiveness of computerized instruction. These two steps would logically lead to a statement of the purpose of the study.

SUMMARY

Selecting a problem, determining its significance or importance, and relating these factors to one's understanding of the purpose of nursing research are all necessary before starting a research project. It is important to remember that the statement of the problem to be studied and the statement of the purpose of the study are not the same. The problem is a broad question that needs to be answered or an unsatisfactory condition for which a solution is sought. The purpose is the specific aim of the study, which may be to describe, to explain, or to predict something related to the problem's solution.

REFERENCES

Beck, C. T. (1994). Replication strategies for nursing research. *Image, 26*(3) 191–194.

Beckstrand, J., & McBride, A. B. (1990). How to form a research interest group. *Nursing Outlook, 38,* 168–171.

Bookbinder, M. (1992). Searching for solutions. *Nursing Spectrum: Greater New York/Tri-State Edition, 4*(13), 10.

Brooten, D., Knapp, H., Borucki, L., Jacobsen, B., Finkler, S., Arnold, L., & Mennuti, M. (1996). Early discharge and home care after unplanned cesarean birth: Nursing care time. *Journal of Obstetric, Gynecologic, and Neonatal Nursing, 25,* 595–600.

Brooten, D., Naylor, M., Brown, L., York. R., Hollingsworth, A., Cohen, S., Roncoli, M., & Jacobsen, B. (1996). Profile of post discharge rehospitalizations and acute care visits for 7 patient groups. *Public Health Nursing, 12,* 128–134.

Brooten, D., Naylor, M., York. R., Brown, L., Roncoli, M., Hollingsworth, A., Cohen, S., Arnold, L., Finkler, S., Munro, B., & Jacobsen, B. (1995). Effects of nurse specialist transitional care on patient outcomes and costs: Results of five randomized trials. *American Journal of Managed Care, 1,* 45–51.

Brown, S. A. (1988). Effects of interventions in diabetes care: A meta-analysis of findings. *Nursing Research, 37,* 223–230.

Brown, S. A. (1990). Quality of reporting in diabetes education research, 1954–1986. *Research in Nursing and Health, 13,* 53–62.

Budin, W. (1998). Psychosocial adjustment to breast cancer in unmarried women. *Research in Nursing and Health, 21,* 155–166.

Engebretson, J. (1996). Comparison of nurses and alternative healers. *Image: Journal of Nursing Scholarship, 28*(2), 95–99.

Feldman, H. R., & Hott, J. R. (1991). Light up your practice with nursing research. *Journal of the New York State Nursing Association, 22,* 8–11.

Humenick, S. (1994). The origin of relevant research questions. *Journal of Perinatal Education, 3*(3), 47.

Kahn, C. (1994). Picking a research problem: The critical decision. *The New England Journal of Medicine, 330*(21), 1530–1533.

Lindeman, C. A. (1975). Priorities in clinical nursing research. *Nursing Outlook, 23,* 693–698.

National Institute of Nursing Research ((NINR). (1993, September 23). *National nursing research agenda: Setting research priorities.* Bethesda, MD: National Institutes of Health.

Redeker, N., Mason, D., Wykpisz, E., & Glica, B. (1996). Sleep patterns in women after coronary artery bypass surgery. *Applied Nursing Research, 9*(3), 115–122.

Rempusheski, V. (1990). Ask an expert. *Applied Nursing Research, 3*(1), 44–46.

Schepp, K. G. (1991). Factors influencing the coping effort of mothers of hospitalized children. *Nursing Research, 40,* 42–46.

Sigma Theta Tau International (1998, January 14). *Online Journal of Knowledge Synthesis for Nursing* [On-line]. Available: http://www.stti.iupui.edu/publications/journal.

Smeltzer, S. C., & Whipple, B. (1991). Women and HIV infection. *Image: Journal of Nursing Scholarship, 23,* 249–256.

Werley, H. H., Fitzpatrick, J. J., Stevenson, J., & Norbeck, J. (Eds.). (1983–present). *Annual review of nursing research.* New York: Springer Publishing Co.

4

The Literature Search

After deciding on the problem to study, there is a need to read more to find out what has already been researched in the area, to get all the ideas necessary to help develop the theoretical framework and hypothesis, and to decide on the research methods to use. The first search of the literature helps you to identify and select a research problem, but the second search should be confined to investigating materials that are directly relevant to the problem to be solved.

A careful, systematic well-organized literature review will include recent publications and will go back as far as is consistent with the nature of the problem chosen for study. It must be sufficiently thorough to familiarize the researcher with past studies pertinent to the one now being planned. For example, Budin (1998) was interested in studying factors related to psychosocial adjustment to breast cancer in unmarried women. A preliminary review of the literature identified the type of surgery, symptom distress, and social support as factors that were related to adjustment in other studies. In planning for her study on adjustment to breast cancer in unmarried women she conducted a comprehensive search of the literature for studies on the effects of mastectomy as compared with breast-conserving surgery, distress resulting from symptoms or side effects of treatment for breast cancer, and the effects of social support on adjustment to serious health conditions and for studies dealing with unmarried women or those women with primary support systems other than the traditional married relationship. In this type of search, each such study found may suggest additional studies to be examined. Another example that illustrates this type of comprehensive literature search is "A Critical Review of Prenatal Attachment Research" (Muller, 1992). Cranley (1992) has prepared a scholarly response to this review that "critiques the critique."

PURPOSE OF THE LITERATURE SEARCH

The purpose of a literature search after you have identified your research question is threefold. One goal will be to gain familiarity with the literature in the field under study. As a researcher, you need to know whether the study planned has already been done. If it has been done, it may bear repeating, or you may decide to study another aspect of the same problem. For example, while Budin was working as a research fellow on a project that investigated patterns of adjustment among breast cancer patients and their partners (Hoskins et al., 1996) she became familiar with the literature on adjustment to breast cancer and decided to focus her research on unmarried women with breast cancer (1998). Her search of the literature showed that although women with supportive husbands seemed to adjust reasonably well, little was know about adjustment in unmarried women. Your second goal is that, if a theoretical framework is used, it must be well-documented and so well-understood that it can be authoritatively related to the study under consideration. Alternative theories should also be reviewed, if they are pertinent, and the reasons given as to why they were not selected. For example, the Gate Control Theory, the most comprehensive model used by researchers to describe the components of pain (Melzack, Belanger, & Lacroix, 1991), is illustrative of a theoretical rationale used by Sittner, Hudson, Grossman, and Gaston-Johansson (1998) in their study of adolescents' perceptions of pain during labor as well as by Whipple and Glynn (1992), who studied the effects of listening to music as a noninvasive method of pain control. Third, the literature review may help you discover various methodologies and measurement tools that might be useful in designing your study.

These purposes may not always prove to be appropriate but may suggest ideas about the method and type of instrument to devise. For example, a questionnaire survey may be the choice eventually made, but there may be no questionnaire in the literature that is tailored to your survey. Therefore, you may decide to set up your own using ideas culled from the literature and from similar types of survey questionnaires. The classic article by Notter (1977), is worth reading to gain a better understanding of "The Significance of the Literature Search in the Research Process." Also recommended is the article by Haller (1988).

Meta-analysis involves merging findings from many studies that have examined the same phenomenon (Burns & Grove, 1997). The use of meta-analysis, an increasingly popular method of interpreting the results of a large number of related studies, may dramatically alter the process of scientific discovery and how the nurse researcher will evaluate individual studies (Footnotes, 1990). Meta-analysis mines the existing cumulative knowledge of the effects of many phenomena and, by averaging together the results of multiple studies, may lessen the importance of individual studies in a literature review. Brown (1988) issues a caveat about the multiplicity of meta-analysis studies and warns that the use has proceeded faster than the development of the statistical theory needed as a basis for meta-analytic procedures, which itself must be tested and substantiated. Nevertheless, reading a study that reports the results of meta-analysis is another way to become familiar with the research literature on a topic. Examples of studies that used meta-analysis include Brown and Grimes (1995), Devine and Reifschneider (1995), and Kinney, Burfitt, Stullenbarger, Rees, and DeBolt (1996). Beck used this technique in several related studies (1995, 1996a, 1996b). Smith and Stullenbarger (1991) provide a prototype that may be used for integrative review and meta-analysis for nursing research, and Duffy (1988) describes meta-analysis as a quantitative approach to synthesizing research findings across studies.

DOCUMENTING THE SEARCH

Every study reviewed in a literature search should be evaluated as to its strengths and limitations, methods used, results obtained, and relevance to the study being planned. A record should be kept on all references reviewed, and each entry should include the complete citation of the reference, that is, author(s) name(s); title of the report, article, or book; name of journal or publisher; date of publication; pages on which the material appears; and the notes you have made on it. Careful note taking and reference citation will save many headaches later when you get into the study and when you prepare the report (Foreman & Kirchhoff, 1987). A computerized record-keeping system may be helpful, or if you are not computer literate, index cards are fine. The key is to be organized and to have a system.

Brown (1990) describes the rigorous process used in evaluating the quality of reporting in diabetes patient education research for the years 1954 to 1986. Employing Duffy's (1985) research appraisal checklist, Brown reviewed bibliographic citations from primary research studies and narrative reviews of diabetic patient teaching and performed computer searches using MEDLINE, Combined Health Information Data Base, Psychological Abstracts, ERIC, and Dissertation Abstracts (for diabetes studies). To identify unpublished master's studies, Brown surveyed 128 NLN-accredited MS graduate degree nursing programs. She also followed-up by seeking information from 26 diabetes training and research centers to locate unpublished as well as published research reports, a difficult area to access. Brown found serious problems with the quality of diabetes patient education research and, sadly, that although nurses may be conducting research, they are not publishing their results.

LOCATING THE RELEVANT LITERATURE

The most important resource for a literature search is a good library. Every nurse should develop skill in the use of this resource. If you need assistance in learning how to make the best use of the library, the reference librarian can be most helpful in explaining the use of card catalogues, indexes, abstracts, directories, and computerized databases, all designed to open doors to the available literature.

Nursing is very fortunate in having a number of important tools that give access to the nursing literature. Abstracts of studies in nursing have appeared in the journal *Nursing Research* since 1959. They covered studies in public health nursing from 1924 to 1978 and other studies in nursing or relevant to nursing from 1955 through 1978. *Nursing Abstracts,* published by Nursing Abstracts Co. Inc. (P. O. Box 295, Forest Hills, NY 11375), is issued quarterly. Henderson's *Nursing Studies Index,* a four-volume annotated index, lists all studies reported during the period from 1900 to 1959. The *Cumulative Index to Nursing and Allied Health Literature* (CINAHL) is an index especially important to nursing. CINAHL, which covers the period from 1956 on, provides authoritative coverage of the professional literature in nursing and 17 allied health disciplines, biomedicine, consumer health, and health science librarianship. Virtually all nursing journals are indexed, along with publications from the ANA and the NLN. CINAHL also provides access to health care books, book chapters, pamphlets, nursing dissertations, selected conference proceedings, audiovisual material, and educational software (CINAHL, 1998). Also recommended are the *International Nursing Index* (INI), which lists worldwide nursing literature from 1966 on and, of course, the annual indexes to the various nursing periodicals. The *Encyclopedia of Nursing Research* (1998), edited by Joyce J. Fitzpatrick, is a mandate for nurse researchers and research students at all levels. This reference clarifies and presents information on the background and development of key nursing research concepts and areas of study.

Computerized searches were once considered the wave of the future, but the future is now, because most university libraries have computers that can be used to access and search a variety of databases. Databases are also available on CD-ROM as well as from home via Internet connections to university libraries. Web-based databases are changing the way students use the library in a world where resources are becoming more and more Internet-based.

Sigma Theta Tau's Virginia Henderson International Nursing Library also offers electronic services that can be tapped into from home and university offices around the world. This outstanding facility, located at the Center for Nursing Scholarship in Indianapolis is a "unique, state-of-the-art computerized facility that provides subscribers access to current nursing research and the opportunity to network globally with nurses and health care professionals" (Sigma Theta Tau International, 1998c). The Virginia Henderson Library also houses the Registry of Nursing Research. This free benefit to Sigma Theta Tau International members since January 1, 1998, is an electronic research resource constructed from data contributed by the nurse researchers themselves. It currently contains almost 10,000 studies. The registry contains biographical data about nurse researchers, their research programs and studies, and the results of their studies, including abstracts and information about related studies (Sigma Theta Tau International, 1998a). In January 1994, the Library launched *The Online Journal of Knowledge Synthesis for Nursing* (Barnsteiner, 1994). This peer-reviewed electronic journal can be accessed virtually 24 hours a day and provides critical reviews of research pertinent to clinical practice and research situations that nurses can access and use immediately. Special features include full-text articles, full-text searches, hypertext navigation, links to CINAHL, MEDLINE, tables, and figures (Sigma Theta Tau International, 1998b). Access to the library services are available via the Sigma Theta Tau International Home Page on the Internet (see appendix E for a listing of helpful Internet web sites and chapter 10 for more on using computers in research).

The nurse researcher may also want to make use of related reference tools in the fields of medicine, biology, sociology, psychology, or education. Particularly helpful are the large electronic databases of Psychological Abstracts (PsychLIT), the Educational Resources Information Center (ERIC), and MEDLINE (Sinclair, 1987). MEDLINE contains citations to more than 9 million articles that have been published in 3,800 biomedical journals, books, technical reports, manuscripts, microfilms, and pictorial materials (MEDLINE, 1998). In 1997, the National Library of Medicine (NLM) announced that it would offer its MEDLINE database free of charge on the World Wide Web. Leading nursing journals currently indexed in INI are included in MEDLINE. Abdellah (1990) describes the NLM as a treasure trove for nurse researchers. For an excellent reference on "Keeping Abreast of the Literature Electronically" see Nicoll (1993) and also Sinclair (1987).

PRIMARY AND SECONDARY SOURCES

When doing a literature search, one must be careful to differentiate between primary and secondary sources. A primary source is a description of research written by the person who actually did the study. A reference to a piece of research by someone other than the original researcher is a secondary source. An abstract is a brief summarization of a research project. Writing an abstract of a study requires a special skill. A well-written abstract tells what was done, how it was done, the results obtained, and how the author interprets the results (New York State Nurses Association, 1996). (See appendix C for guidelines on writing a research abstract). Although published abstracts of studies and integrative reviews of the literature are important as a way of locating relevant studies, they should not be cited as primary sources because information contained in abstracts or other secondary sources are often summarized and may include interpretations by the abstractor or even inaccuracies. To be sure of the facts and to be able to draw your own conclusions, you need to read the original, or primary, source.

Differentiation between primary and secondary sources is of vital importance in historical research. In documenting primary resources one must examine the actual records, rather than the secondary accounts of what is in the records. For example, a researcher who quotes Florence Nightingale from the original "Notes on Nursing: What It Is and What It Is Not" (Nightingale, 1859) is using a primary source. If a similar quote is taken from a passage published in "Notes on Nursing Science" (The Nightingale Society, 1998), the author is using a secondary source. Using primary sources is equally important in the literature search in descriptive and experimental studies, each of which has its documentation stage, that is, the literature review. Examples of nursing journals that contain a majority of primary sources include *Nursing Research, Research in Nursing and Health, Applied Nursing Research, Western Journal of Nursing Research,* and *Scholarly Inquiry for Nursing* (see appendix D).

RELATIONSHIP OF SEARCH TO RATIONALE

The importance of identifying the significance of the study for nursing was mentioned in the preceding chapter. The literature search should contribute to the argument for the importance of the investigation. Information gleaned from the literature should help to delineate the boundaries of the problem more clearly, to discuss it in relation to previous studies and show how it differs from others, and to indicate how this study is expected to add to our knowledge and improve our practice.

The search may also unearth theories related to the solution of the problem. Therefore, it is important to be on the lookout for those that offer promising explanations for the phenomenon under study. Whipple, Ogden, and Komisaruk (1992), for example, offer physiological and psychological theories relating to pain threshold, analgesia, and genital self-stimulation in women, making extensive use of documented research to develop their scientific rationale.

THE THEORETICAL FRAMEWORK

The review of the literature may embrace broad areas of content related to the problem the investigator plans to study. Eventually, however, the content covered must be evaluated and the body of knowledge that is clearly focused on the approach selected for the study planned identified. Those theories or concepts that offer a promising approach to the study planned and selected as guiding the study are known as the theoretical framework; they are sometimes called the conceptual framework.

In the past, most nursing research was characterized by a lack of a theoretical or conceptual framework (Batey, 1977; Ellis, 1977). Often, there was no attempt to identify and present concepts or theories useful in guiding the study. Sometimes a "framework" consisted of a listing of facts with little or no effort to relate these as a rationale for the study and no effort later to discuss the study findings in relation to them. Brown (1990) and Beck (1990) emphasize the need to critically assess research for its relationship to a theoretical or conceptual rationale and also the definitions of the constructs under examination.

In the controversial arena surrounding estrogen replacement therapy (ERT), Logothetis (1991) uses a health belief model (HBM) as a framework to understand women's decisions about ERT. Woods, Taylor, Mitchell, and Lentz (1992) use a variation of a similar conceptual framework, the concept of health-seeking behavior, to help account for perimenstrual symptoms. Sherman (1996) used Rogers' (1992) framework of the science of unitary human beings to examine relationships among spirituality, perceived social support, death anxiety, and nurses' willingness to care for AIDS patients. Budin (1998) used a framework guided by concepts and propositions derived from the theoretical and empirical literature on stress, social support, and adjustment to illness to hypothesize that stressors associated with primary treatment alternatives; variability in appraisal of the stressful nature of breast cancer treatments, conceptualized as symptom distress; and the presence of interpersonal resources within the social environment, conceptualized as perceived social support, would account for a significant proportion of the variance in psychosocial adjustment to breast cancer. For a more extensive explanation of the relationship of theory and research, see Fawcett and Downs (1992).

SUMMARY

The literature review required before undertaking a research project is somewhat like the work of a detective, and it can be equally fascinating. Each new find becomes more exciting than the last, especially if it brings new understanding of the problem or an idea for the research method that might be employed.

Although the researcher tries to limit reading to relevant topics, it is also possible to have the delightful intellectual experience of getting off the main path and being lured onto interesting bypaths. If you suddenly find yourself reading something that has captured your interest but that has absolutely nothing to do with your study, do not be surprised. Enjoy the detour. This is not an uncommon experience. It may even lead to the serendipitous identification of other problems you will want to study later. Such seductive flirtations should be kept to a minimum, however, and self-discipline may be needed at times to keep your focus on your main concern—the literature that is relevant to your current study.

If your reading is well directed, you will come up with a carefully thought out problem that is related to the research in the area and, if pertinent, with a theory or concepts that can be tested by your study. If your work is well done, you will be ready for the next step, the development of a hypothesis to be tested.

REFERENCES

Abdellah, F. (1990). The National Library of Medicine—a treasure trove for nurse researchers. *Journal of Professional Nursing, 6,* 134.

Barnsteiner, J. (1994). The Online Journal of Knowledge Synthesis for Nursing. *Reflections, 20*(2), 10–11.

Batey, M. V. (1977). Conceptualization: Knowledge and logic guiding empirical research. *Nursing Research, 26,* 324–329.

Beck, C. T. (1990). The research critique. *Journal of Obstetric, Gynecologic and Neonatal Nursing, 19,* 18–22.

Beck, C. T. (1995). The effects of postpartum depression on maternal-infant interaction: A meta-analysis. *Nursing Research, 44,* 298–304.

Beck, C. T. (1996a). A meta-analysis of the relationship between postpartum depression and infant temperament. *Nursing Research, 45*(4), 225–230.

Beck, C. T. (1996b). A meta-analysis of predictors of postpartum depression. *Nursing Research, 45*(5), 297–303.

Brown, S., & Grimes, D. (1995). A meta-analysis of nurse practitioners and nurse midwives in primary care. *Nursing Research, 44*(6), 332–339.

Brown, S. A. (1988). Effects of interventions in diabetes and care: A meta-analysis of findings. *Nursing Research, 37,* 223–230.

Brown, S. A. (1990). Quality of reporting in diabetes patient education research: 1954–1986. *Research in Nursing and Health, 13,* 53–62.

Budin, W. (1998). Psychosocial adjustment to breast cancer in unmarried women. *Research in Nursing and Health, 21,* 155–166.

Burns, N., & Grove, S. (1997). *The practice of nursing research: Conduct, critique, & utilization.* Philadelphia: W. B. Saunders Co.

CINAHL. (1998, January 14). *CINAHL Information Systems for Nursing and Allied Health* [On-line]. Available: http://www.cinahl.com.

Cranley, M. S. (1992). Response to "A critical review of pre-natal attachment research." *Scholarly Inquiry for Nursing Practice, 6,* 23–26.

Cumulative Index to Nursing and Allied Health Literature (CINAHL). (1977–present). Glendale, CA: Glendale Adventist Medical Center.

Devine, E., & Reifschneider, E. (1995). A meta-analysis of the effects of psychoeducational care in adults with hypertension. *Nursing Research, 44*(4), 237–245.

Duffy, M. E. (1985). A research appraisal checklist for evaluating nursing research reports. *Nursing and Healthcare, 6,* 539–547.

Duffy, M. E. (1988). Meta-analysis: A quantitative approach to synthesizing research findings across studies. *Nursing and Healthcare, 11,* 287–289.

Ellis, R. (1977). Fallibilities, fragments, and frames. *Nursing Research, 26,* 177–182.

Fawcett, J., & Downs, F. S. (1992). *The relationship of theory and research* (2nd ed.). East Norwalk, CT: Appleton & Lange.

Fitzpatrick, J. (1998). *Encyclopedia of nursing research.* New York: Springer Publishing Co.

Footnotes (1990, July 11). *Chronicle of Higher Education,* A4.

Foreman, M., & Kirchhoff, K. (1987). Accuracy of references in nursing journals. *Research in Nursing and Health, 10,* 177–183.

Haller, K. B. (1988). Conducting a literature review. *Maternal Child Nursing, 13,* 148.

Henderson, V., et al. (1963, 1966, 1970, 1972). *Nursing Studies Index* (Vols. 1–4, 1900–1959). Philadelphia: Lippincott. Vol. 1, 1972; Vol. 2, 1970; Vol. 3, 1966; Vol. 4, 1963. (Vol. 1 covers the period 1900 to 1929; Vol. 2, the period 1930 to 1949; Vol. 3, the period 1950 to 1956; Vol. 4, the period 1957 to 1959.)

Hoskins, C., Baker, S., Sherman, D., Bohlander, J., Bookbinder, M., Budin, W., Ekstrom, D., Knauer, C., & Maislin, G. (1996). Social support and patterns of adjustment to breast cancer. *Scholarly Inquiry for Nursing Practice: An International Journal, 10*(2), 99–123.

International Nursing Index (INI). (1966–present). New York: American Journal of Nursing Company.

Kinney, M., Burfitt, S., Stullenbarger, E., Rees, B., & DeBolt, M. (1996). Quality of life in cardiac patient research: A meta-analysis. *Nursing Research, 45*(3), 173–180.

Logothetis, M. L. (1991). Women's decisions about estrogen replacement therapy. *Western Journal of Nursing Research, 13,* 458–474.

MEDLINE. (1998, January 14). *Free Medline: PubMed and Internet Grateful Med.* [On-line]. Available: http://www.nlm.nih.gov/databases/freemedl.html.

Melzack, R, Belanger, E., & Lacroix, R. (1991). Effect of maternal position on front and back pain. *Journal of Pain and Symptom Management, 6,* 476–480.

Muller, M. E. (1992). A critical review of pre-natal attachment research. *Scholarly Inquiry for Nursing Practice, 6,* 5–22.

New York State Nurses Association. (1996). Writing a research abstract. In *A compendium of articles, position statements, and related materials to advance nursing research in New York State.* New York: Author.

Nicoll, L. (1993) Keeping abreast of the literature electronically. *Nursing Research, 42*(5), 315–317.

Nightingale, F. (1859). *Notes on nursing: what it is and what it is not.* London: Harrison, 59, Pall Mall. Reproduced by offset in 1946 by Edward Stern & Co., Philadelphia.

The Nightingale Society. (1998). Notes on nursing science. Carmel, CA: *Nightingale Society, 10*(4) 2–4.

Notter, L. E. (1977). The significance of the literature search in the research process. In ANA, *Reference resources for research and continuing education* (pp. 25–30). Kansas City, MO: American Nurses Association.

Nursing Abstracts Co. Inc. P. O. Box 295, Forest Hills, NY 11375.

Rogers, M. (1992). Nursing science and the space age. *Nursing Science Quarterly, 5*(1), 27–34.

Sherman, D. (1996). Nurses' willingness to care for AIDS patients and spirituality, social support, and death anxiety. *Image, 28*(3), 205–213.

Sigma Theta Tau International (1998a, January 14). *About Sigma Theta Tau International Registry of Nursing Research* [On-line]. Available: http://www.stti.iupui.edu/rnr/.

Sigma Theta Tau International (1998b, January 14). STTI Publications: *Online Journal of Knowledge Synthesis for Nursing* [On-line]. Available: http://www.stti.iupui.edu/publications/journal/.

Sigma Theta Tau International (1998c, January 14). *Virginia Henderson International Library* [On-line]. Available: http://www.stti.iupui.edu/library.

Sinclair, V. (1987). Literature searches by computer. *Image, 19,* 35–37.

Sittner, B., Hudson, D., Grossman, C., & Gaston-Johansson, F. (1998). Adolescents' perceptions of pain during labor. *Clinical Nursing Research, 7*(1), 82–93.

Smith, M., & Stullenbarger, E. (1991). A prototype for integrative review and meta-analysis for nursing research. *Journal of Advanced Nursing, 16*(11), 1272–1283.

Whipple, B., & Glynn, N. J. (1992). Quantification of the effects of listening to music as a noninvasive method of pain control. *Scholarly Inquiry for Nursing Practice, 6,* 43–58.

Whipple, B., Ogden, G., & Komisaruk, B. R. (1992). Physiological correlates of imagery-induced orgasm in women. *Archives of Sexual Behavior, 21,* 121–133.

Woods, N. F., Taylor, D., Mitchell, E. S., & Lentz, M. J. (1992). Perimenstrual symptoms and health-seeking behavior. *Western Journal of Nursing Research, 14,* 418–443.

5

The Hypothesis

Some research studies involve the development and testing of hypotheses. Hypothesis development and testing models of research are most often specific to quantitative research. A hypothesis is a statement of the predicted relationships between the factors one wishes to analyze, that is, the variables in a study. The hypothesis grows out of the problem to be studied and the theoretical framework that has been developed for the study. It is a tentative solution or explanation of the problem that the investigator has arrived at through a review of the literature, in other words, a theory you have found that appears to explain the situation or one you have developed on the basis of your own experience.

Thus, it is apparent that hypotheses are not just guesses. They may be based on hunches in the beginning, but by the time the study actually gets under way these hunches are educated hunches and have been refined into a carefully thought out statement of the problem supported by a rationale based on a careful review of the relevant literature.

PURPOSE OF THE HYPOTHESIS

That formulating the hypothesis is a very important step in any research project becomes evident when we consider that the hypothesis determines the type of study that will be done and the variables that will be studied. An examination of the following three hypotheses, proposed by Rentschler (1991) in her study of the correlates of successful breast-feeding, will show this relationship. The hypotheses tested were as follows:

1. There would be a positive relationship between pregnant women's achievement motivation and success in breast-feeding.
2. There would be a positive relationship between pregnant women's level of information about breast-feeding and success in breast-feeding.

3. When taken together, the variables of pregnant women's achievement motivation and information about breast-feeding would be better predictors of success in breast-feeding than either one taken alone (Rentschler, 1991, p. 152).

These hypotheses identify (1) the population that will be studied: pregnant women who planned to breast-feed; (2) the problem solutions that have been selected for successful breast-feeding: achievement motivation and information about breast-feeding; (3) the dependent and independent variables to be studied: successful breast-feeding (for at least 6 weeks), measured by Rentschler's Breastfeeding Experience Questionnaire (BEQ) (1986) and her Personal Data Inventory (1986); and (4) the measurements to be used for the independent variables, achievement motivation, measured by a Questionnaire Measure of Individual Differences in Achieving Tendency (QMIDAT) (Mehrabian & Bank, 1978), and information about breast-feeding, measured by the Gulick (1981) Information on Breastfeeding Questionnaire (IBQ).

It should be noted that these hypotheses flowed directly from the description of the problem: what makes the difference in the outcome for women who attempt to breast-feed? In this study, all the hypotheses positively predicted the results the nurse researcher expected to obtain.

Such a prediction does not indicate a bias on the part of the investigator; it simply provides a framework for the study. The design of the study must preserve the objectivity of the experiment, and the results will permit either support or nonsupport of the hypotheses.

The following study was an excellent example of how predictions about the nature of the relationship of variables were explored in another study. Miller and Perry (1990) used a two-group pretest and posttest quasi-experimental design to determine the effectiveness of a slow, deep-breathing relaxation technique in relieving postoperative pain after CABG surgery. Their hypotheses included the following:

1. Patients after CABG surgery who are taught and use a relaxation technique will have a greater decrease in vital signs after using the technique than those who do not.
2. Patients after CABG surgery who are taught and use a relaxation technique will have a greater perception of pain than those who are not taught, as indicated by a self-report of pain on a visual analogue scale (VAS).
3. Patients after CABG surgery who are taught and use a relaxation technique will have a greater decrease in perception of pain than those not taught this technique, as indicated by self-report on a visual descriptor scale (VDS).

4. Patients after CABG surgery who are taught a relaxation technique will require fewer analgesics in a 24-hour period after extubation than those not taught the technique (Miller & Perry, 1990, p. 145).

Although hypotheses 1 and 3 were supported in this study and 2 and 4 were not, the nursing implications indicate the possible benefits of incorporating relaxation techniques in the postoperative period for the purpose of pain reduction.

Some investigators use what is known as the null hypothesis. Instead of predicting a significant difference or relationship between the independent variable and the dependent variables (see chapter 6), they predict no significant difference or relationship. The null hypothesis is related to the statistical test to be used (see chapter 8). Rejection of the null hypothesis allows the researcher to accept the alternative: that there is a significant difference between the groups or a significant relationship between the variables examined.

THEORETICAL FRAMEWORK AND THE HYPOTHESIS

Not only does the nature of the problem influence the hypothesis, but the theoretical framework of the study also is directly related to it. In the Miller and Perry (1990) study cited previously, present pain theories underlie their hypotheses (p. 137). Rentschler (1991) used achievement motivation theory and theories about expectancy of success and the value of incentive as the rationale for her hypotheses.

Sherman (1996) used Martha Rogers' (1970, 1992) Science of Unitary Human Beings as a theoretical framework to investigate the willingness of nurses to care for AIDS patients. Describing how this framework guides this study, Sherman explains,

> Within the Rogerian framework, the AIDS epidemic may be viewed as an example of human-environmental diversity that demands courage, risk-taking and compassion (Rogers, 1992). The science of unitary human beings offers a paradigm from which one can derive theories that describe a phenomenon of concern, such as nurses' willingness to care for AIDS patients. In this study, it was theorized that a person's experiences and awareness of integrality with the environment promotes a conceptualization of self beyond a physical dimension, infinite with the universe, and supports the view of death not as an end state but as a transition into life ever new (Reeder, 1990). People thus find meaning in life and death, enhancing their capacity to participate in change by exercising choices in fulfillment of their potential (Rogers, 1970). The experience

> and awareness of human-environmental integrality was conceptualized as spirituality and perceived social support. The interpretation of death was conceptualized as death anxiety. It was hypothesized that spirituality, perceived social support, and death anxiety would be related to a nurse's choice in fulfilling nursing potential, made evident by a willingness to care for AIDS patients. (Sherman, 1996, pp. 205–206)

A refereed journal, *Visions: The Journal of Rogerian Nursing Science,* published by the Society of Rogerian Scholars, Inc., features studies that use Rogers' theories. For other examples of how this theorist's Science of Unitary Human Beings is used in current research, see *Rogerian Nursing Science News, the Newsletter of the Society of Rogerian Scholars, Inc.*

Yes, the use of theory can be an important technique in developing a conceptual framework for a study, and this conceptual framework will, in turn, influence the nature of the hypothesis and its relation to the total study.

IS A HYPOTHESIS ALWAYS NECESSARY?

Although formulating the hypothesis is a necessary step in explanatory or experimental research, it may or may not be required in descriptive research. Some descriptive studies are exploratory in nature and may actually be done in order to generate hypotheses.

The following is an example of a study that raises questions rather than stating hypotheses. Lindgren, Burke, Hainsworth, and Eakes (1992) explore, in a very sensitive, perceptive way, the concept of chronic sorrow. They raise major research questions about the differences and similarities of chronic sorrow, resolvable grief, and depression that need to be examined in a variety of populations before a conceptual framework can be built and hypotheses generated. Questions include the following:

1. Does chronic sorrow occur in a variety of populations across the life span?
2. What are the characteristics of chronic sorrow in these populations?
3. How does the expression of chronic sorrow in these populations compare with the chronic sorrow experienced by parents of children with disabilities?
4. Is chronic sorrow an inherent phenomenon in chronic illness situations? Each of these questions could lead to important areas for future study (Lindgren et al., 1992, p. 38).

Some studies may test hypotheses and ask research questions. For example, Budin (1998) hypothesized that there would be significant relationships among primary treatment alternatives, symptom distress, perceived social support, and psychosocial adjustment to breast cancer in unmarried women. Since little was known about the social support network structure of unmarried women dealing with early treatment for breast cancer, the following research questions were also posed:

1. Who are the primary sources of social support identified by unmarried women experiencing treatment for breast cancer?
2. Do levels of perceived social support vary among sources?

Another type of investigation that does not require the statement of a hypothesis is one that is done primarily to test a research instrument. Such a study is necessary when there are no known tested instruments that can be used for investigating a particular problem or when existing instruments have not been validated with specific populations because the use of an untested or invalidated instrument may well create lack of confidence in the study findings.

Hill and Humenick (1996) describe the development and testing of the psychometric properties of a new instrument, the H & H Lactation Scale. This instrument was examined in studies using two separate samples, mothers of low birth weight infants and mothers of term infants. The conceptual framework of insufficient milk supply (IMS) proposed by Hill and Humenick served as a guide for the development of items in both studies. This framework focuses on direct and indirect antecedents that may influence the mother's perception of insufficient milk. The items for the H & H Lactation Scale were developed for the purpose of measuring the IMS indicators, and subscales identified by factor analysis measured three concepts: maternal confidence or commitment to breast-feeding, perceived infant breast-feeding satiety, and maternal-infant breast-feeding satisfaction.

England and Roberts (1996) also report a study designed to establish the validity and reliability of a new instrument, the Parent Caregiver Strain Questionnaire (PCSQ). This instrument was developed in response to the need for a valid and reliable way to measure the antecedents and consequences of caregiving events as well as the caregiving events themselves. Factor analysis was performed with data from 283 adult children who were providing care to a neurologically impaired patient, and it revealed five well-defined factors. The findings from this study provide beginning evidence of the adequacy of the PCSQ and suggest that for adult offspring, caregiver strain is a multidimensional response to the burdens of caregiving.

Champion and Scott's 1997 study "Reliability and Validity of Breast Cancer Screening Belief Scales in African American Women" is an example of instrument testing with a specific population. The investigators documented the need to develop culturally sensitive scales to measure beliefs related to mammography and breast self-examination (BSE) screening. Although breast cancer incidence is higher among White women, African American women have a higher mortality rate from this disease, and few African American women have mammogram. So that research information may be maximally applied to understanding breast screening beliefs in African American women, it is imperative that culturally sensitive, reliable, and valid measures be used for data collection.

After the instrument has met the criteria of validity and reliability, the investigator can move on to the next stage of the research, the testing of the hypothesis. In this case, Champion and Scott (1997) hypothesized that breast cancer screening behaviors would be related to perceived susceptibility to breast cancer. It was further hypothesized that benefits and barriers to mammography screening would be correlated with mammography compliance and that benefits and barriers to BSE would also be related to BSE behaviors.

SUMMARY

We have given considerable attention to the hypothesis because of its great importance in an investigator's preparation for some quantitative studies. The following chapter, which deals with research method, will bring out the close relationship of the hypothesis to the research method used.

REFERENCES

Budin, W. (1998). Psychosocial adjustment to breast cancer in unmarried women. *Research in Nursing and Health, 21,* 155–166.

Champion, V., & Scott, C. (1997). Reliability and validity of breast cancer screening belief scales in African American women. *Nursing Research, 46,* 331–337.

England, M., & Roberts, B. (1996). Theoretical and psychometric analysis of caregiver strain. *Research in Nursing and Health, 19,* 499–510.

Gulick, E. E. (1981). The relationship between expectant mothers' sex role orientation, nurturance, maternal attitudes, information on breast-feeding, and successful breast-feeding. *Dissertation Abstracts International, 37*(02), 567B. (University Microfilms No. 8115-493)

Hill, P., & Humenick, S. (1996). Development of the H & H Lactation Scale. *Nursing Research, 45,* 136–140.

Lindgren, C. L., Burke, M. L., Hainsworth, M. A., & Eakes, G. G. (1992). Chronic sorrow, a lifespan concept. *Scholarly Inquiry for Nursing Practice, 6,* 27–40.

Mehrabian, A., & Bank, L. (1978). A questionnaire measure of individual differences in achieving tendency. *Educational and Psychological Measurements, 38,* 47.

Miller, K. M., & Perry, P. A. (1990). Relaxation techniques and postoperative pain in patients undergoing cardiac surgery. *Heart and Lung, 19,* 136–146.

Reeder, F. (1990). Forward. In E.A.M. Barrett (Ed.), *Visions of Rogers' science-based nursing* (p. xix). New York: National League of Nursing.

Rentschler, D. D. (1986). The relationship between pregnant women's achievement motivation, information about breast-feeding, and successful breast-feeding. *Dissertation Abstracts International,* 47, 4114B. (University Microfilms No. 8625-650)

Rentschler, D. D. (1991). Correlates of successful breast-feeding. *Image: Journal of Nursing Scholarship, 23,* 151–154.

Rogers, M. E. (1970). *An introduction to the theoretical basis of nursing.* Philadelphia: F. A. Davis

Rogers, M. E. (1992). Nursing science and the space age. *Nursing Science Quarterly, 5*(1), 27–34.

Rogerian Nursing Science News. (1992). V, 1–8. (Society of Rogerian Scholars, Canal Street Station, P. O. Box 1195, New York, NY 10013-9793.)

Sherman, D. (1996). Nurses' willingness to care for AIDS patients and spirituality, social support, and death anxiety. *Image, 28*(3), 205–213.

6

The Research Method

Once you have selected the problem you wish to study, systematically reviewed the related literature, and developed the questions or hypothesis based on logical rationale and a theoretical framework, you are ready to begin work on the design for the study. Think of the design as a blueprint that will guide your work. Too often the researcher selects the method first and does not attend to the total process of selection based on the research question. Identifying the type of problem to be solved and stating the purpose of the study will reveal whether the study will be an exploratory, descriptive, correlational, or experimental study and thus will dictate the use of either qualitative or quantitative research methods.

QUANTITATIVE METHODS

For any discussion of quantitative research method to be meaningful to the neophyte, certain frequently used terms need to be defined. For example, the terms *independent variable* and *dependent variable* are commonly used in experimental designs and may be mentioned in some quantitative descriptive studies. A *variable* is any factor, characteristic, quality, or attribute under study. An independent variable is one that the investigator manipulates or introduces into the situation; it is also sometimes called the manipulated variable. A dependent variable is one that is under observation by the investigator in order to note what effect the introduction of an independent variable has on it; it is the terminal outcome or behavior and is sometimes called the criterion variable. In the Miller and Perry (1990) study discussed in chapter 5, the independent or manipulated variable was a slow, rhythmic, deep-breathing technique and conversation. The experimenters introduced the variable of structured teaching, in order to compare the results with conversation alone. The dependent variable was postoperative pain, estimated by blood pressure, heart rate, respiratory rate, visual analog scores (VAS), visual descriptor scale (VDS) scores, and analgesic use.

Often, other variables in an experiment will need to be controlled. These are called *control variables* or extraneous variables. Unless these variables are controlled or held constant, they intervene and confound the results, making it hard to know whether the independent variable or one of these extraneous intervening variables caused the effect found. For example, in the Miller and Perry (1990) study, certain controls were established for the selection of subjects in order to exclude extraneous variables: previous CABG surgery, chronic pain, diagnosis of cancer, preoperative or postoperative complications, presence of an intra-aortic balloon pump, extubation time of more than 8 hours postoperative, pulmonary edema, return to operating room, cardiogenic shock, cardiac arrest, unconsciousness, or death (p. 139). In other situations, the time of day that observations are made may be important or, as would be the case in the study of environment on body site temperature in full-term neonates, the temperature of the room or environment (Cusson, Madonia, & Taekman, 1997).

You can probably think of a number of other variables that may be important to control in certain studies. In any event, it is always wise to try to equate the control variables in the experimental and the control groups in order to make sure you are free to concentrate on the independent and dependent variables in the study. Zeller, Good, Cranston-Anderson, and Zeller (1997) address this issue in their interesting article.

Variables are usually defined conceptually and operationally. A *conceptual definition* provides the reader with a clear description of the meaning of the variable. It is similar to a dictionary definition. An *operational definition* explains how a variable is observed or measured. A criterion measure is a characteristic quality or attribute that can be used to measure the effect of the independent variable on the subjects studied. For example, in the study that compared the abdomen, thigh, and arm as sites for subcutaneous sodium heparin injections (Fahs & Kinney, 1991), one of the criterion measures was bruising. A bruise in this study was conceptually defined as "soft tissue injuries resulting from the trauma of subcutaneous injections of heparin." A bruise was operationally defined as "a discolored, purpuric lesion that will change color and fade over a period of time, however, it will not blanch with pressure." The size of each bruise was measured by two methods. The first method was a measurement of the widest diameter directly on the skin. The second method was a trace of the outline of the bruise onto a piece of polyethylene wrap with a fine ball-point pen. The outline was then traced onto a graph with the use of carbon paper and later used to calculate the surface area in square millimeters. A clear operational definition allows for replication by providing the reader with the exact steps or operations that were used to measure the variable.

Some simple, easy-to-apply criterion measures are temperature, blood pressure, and inches in length. Those that involve abstract concepts are sometimes more difficult to apply. For example, in the Rentschler study (1991) the outcome variable successful breast-feeding (defined as breast-feeding for at least 6 weeks) was measured by Rentschler's (1986) BEQ and her Personal Data Inventory (1986). Errors or variations can occur, however, in even so simple a task as taking the patient's temperature (Flo & Brown, 1995). Hence, careful investigators make every effort to ensure accuracy of measurement. They make sure that everyone who is responsible for taking measurements or making observations in the study has been carefully instructed in the technique to be used. Also, if more than one observer or rater is involved, checks are made on how much agreement exists between their observations or ratings. Although perfection is not the goal, the investigator is looking for high interrater or interobserver agreement and reliability (see chapter 7 for more on measurement).

THE DESCRIPTIVE STUDY DESIGN

The descriptive design is the most common type of quantitative study used in nursing research. For example, Redeker, Mason, Wykpisz, and Glica (1996), whose descriptive study was mentioned in chapter 3, wanted to describe sleep patterns in women after CABG surgery. They presented no hypothesis; in essence, their research questions were: What are the changes in day, evening, night, and total daily sleep in women during the first postoperative week and the second posthospitalization week after CABG? What are the changes in day, evening, night, and total daily sleep between the 1st postoperative week (T1), the 1st posthospitalization week (T2), the 6th postoperative week (T3), and the 24th postoperative week (6th month) (T4)? What are the changes in self-reports of sleep behaviors from T1 through T4?

Next, in order to collect the desired data on the sleep patterns of the patients studied, the researchers needed to find an objective, practical, easy-to-use, valid, and reliable instrument. After careful review of the literature on measurement of activity the researchers decided to use the Mini-Motion logger as an instrument to measure sleep. This battery-operated wrist-worn actigraph is an electronic accelerometer that senses motion and has been found to be a valid and reliable measure of sleep patterns (Mason & Redeker, 1993; Mason & Tapp, 1992). The

Sleep-Rest subscale of the Sickness Impact Profile (Bergner, Bobbitt, Carter, & Gilson, 1981) was also used along with the actigraph to measure the impact of illness on behavioral indicators of sleep and rest. Using data collected from a sample of 22 women recovering from CABG, the researchers concluded that nighttime sleep became less fragmented, and, over time, total sleep became more consolidated during nighttime hours, as shown by significant decreases in day, evening, and total sleep and increases in the percentage of total sleep occurring at night. Decreases in the Sleep-Rest subscale indicated perceived improvement in sleep consistent with changes in objective sleep measures over 6 months. These descriptive data can be used to help women anticipate changes in sleep patterns over the course of recovery from CABG surgery.

The purpose of the descriptive correlational study by Jackson, Taylor, and Pyngolil (1991) was to evaluate the relationship among the variables, climacteric status, and physical and mental health symptoms across age cohorts in African American women age 25 to 75 ($N = 522$). They collected their data through home interviews, finding an overall direct relationship between climacteric status and physical health symptoms but not with mental health symptoms. A direct relationship was found between climacteric status and both physical and mental health symptoms in the younger prematurely menopausal cohort (25 to 34), but the cohort of ages 35 to 44 had a direct relationship with their climacteric status and physical health but not with mental health. The study is also interesting because it questioned whether the norms of menopausal studies on Caucasian women could validly be applied to all racial and ethnic groups. It is important for nurse researchers to be aware that findings on male subjects cannot be generalized to females, nor across racial or ethnic groups.

An example of a longitudinal descriptive study was reported by Hoskins et al. (1996a, 1996b). These researchers studied patterns of adjustment among breast cancer patients and their partners over the course of 1 year post surgery. Data were collected at 7 to 10 days; at 1, 2, 3, and 6 months; and at 1 year post surgery. At each data-collection point, the respondents completed four standardized inventories that assessed various dimensions of support and physical and emotional adjustment. The longitudinal design permitted the examination of two different types of questions: (a) the relations between the predictors (marital support and support from other adults) and outcomes (physical and emotional adjustment) at each phase of treatment, considered separately, and (b) the changes over time. Findings indicated that the profound psychosocial impact of breast cancer affects both the woman and her partner, often extending beyond the course of active medical treatment. Four phases of emotional and physical adjustment were identified from the data: diagnosis, post surgery, adjuvant therapy, and ongoing recovery. Women with breast cancer and their partners experienced similar and yet different needs along the diagnostic, treatment, and recovery trajectory. Findings indicated the enormous importance of education, effective communication, support, and other interventions in the interest of promoting psychosocial adjustment in both the woman and her partner(s) over time. Although either a longitudinal or a cross-sectional type of design may be used to study change over a period of time, the longitudinal design, in this situation, was both appropriate and feasible for studying patterns of adjustment to breast cancer in women and their partners.

Although the longitudinal design is useful for studying changes over time, loss of participants through attrition poses a serious threat to the validity of the findings when this method is used. Givin, Keilman, Collins, and Givin (1990) provide useful strategies to minimize attrition in longitudinal studies. These strategies include communication with subjects, preparation of data collectors, facilitating bonding with the study, access and continuity of subject contact with data collectors, showing respect for subjects' time, assuring subjects of the adequacy of their skills and importance of their contribution, and expressing appreciation. Salyer, Geddes, Smith, and Marks (1998) describe how these seven strategies were used to minimize attrition in the Outcomes Research in Nursing Administration (ORNA) Project, a federally funded longitudinal study that examines the relationship among hospital characteristics, nursing unit characteristics, and nursing unit organizational structure, with both patient outcomes and administrative outcomes.

Sometimes a longitudinal design is not feasible because of the time involved, and as a result the sample that is selected cuts across the time periods. For example, if an investigator wished to observe changes in students' risk-taking behaviors, such as sexual intercourse, during the middle school years, the investigator might employ a cross-sectional survey and observe students at each grade of middle school rather than following students in one group through their entire education. A comparative study of "Pathways of influence on fifth and eighth graders' reports about having had sexual intercourse" (Porter, Oakley, Ronis, & Neal, 1996) provides a case in point. The investigators assumed that the use of fifth graders and eighth graders would result in findings that would, for all practical purposes, be as useful as those that would result from a study that followed the students through their middle school experience. Practical decisions of this kind often need to be made, but when they are, the investigators must take into consideration the possible presence of uncontrolled intervening factors that will influence the outcome.

A descriptive survey can be comparative or evaluative in nature. Van Serellen, Lewis, and Leaka (1990) compared stressors affecting adult males hospitalized with the complications of AIDS who were treated on an AIDS special care unit exclusively devoted to their treatment, with stressors affecting a similar group treated on an integrated unit. In comparing the data from structured face-to-face interviews, with 280 from four AIDS special care units and 90 from five integrated units ($N = 370$), the researchers found that, overall, men hospitalized for AIDS complications on units specific to their care experienced fewer stressors compared with their counterparts on integrated units.

Evaluating how much knowledge and understanding college students ($N = 144$) in one large university had of health risks after reading an article in the popular press, Yeaton, Smith, and Rogers (1990) concluded that health care promoters need to be alerted to how conflicting, confusing, and often misleading and distorted media reporting can be, and that age, educational level, race, and health status may play salient roles in readers' and viewers' interpretations of health data in the media.

THE EXPERIMENTAL STUDY DESIGN

In contrast to the descriptive study, which deals with "what is," and the historical study, which examines "what was," experimental research is interested in predicting something in the future. Something new is introduced into a situation, and appropriate quantitative methods are used to determine or measure its effect on the situation. In order to control the situation to the extent possible, the experimental design calls for at least an experimental and a control group. To control for bias, subjects are randomly assigned to these groups.

In the Miller and Perry (1990) study the intensive care unit that was used had four patients in each room, and the investigator could not control postoperative room assignment. Random assignment to experimental or control conditions could have resulted in these subjects being in the same room. To solve this, all subjects in the same week were assigned to the same condition, with the condition for week 1 randomly assigned, and the experimental and control conditions systematically determined thereafter. In a double-blind study, bias is further controlled by seeing that the individual responsible for measuring the results does not know which subjects are in the control group and which are in the experimental group. Both groups are tested before and after the independent variable is introduced to the experimental group. To rule out changes that may occur in both groups as a reaction to the pretest or simply because of intervening experiences or the passage of time, a third group (the second control group) is added. This third group is posttested only.

The "true" experimental design described by Campbell and Stanley (1963) requires manipulation of an independent variable, random assignment to groups, and control over the situation. A design with these features was followed by Vessey, Carlson, and McGill (1994) in their study. These researchers hypothesized that children receiving a distraction intervention would report less pain and display less behavioral distress after venipuncture than children not receiving the distraction intervention would. Children were randomly assigned to an experimental or control group. During venipuncture, the control subjects received standard preparation, which consisted of being comforted by physical touch and soft voices; experimental subjects were encouraged to use a kaleidoscope as a distraction technique. Perception of pain was measured with the Wong-Baker FACES Pain Rating Scale (Wong & Baker, 1988). This instrument consists of a series of six faces that range from very happy to very sad and tearful placed horizontally on a piece of paper. The instrument is treated as a Likert scale with scores ranging from 0 (very happy) to 5 (tearful). (See Figure 7.2, p. 107, for an example of the FACES scale.) A behavioral observation tool was also used to rate the child's intensity of pain on six verbal and motor behaviors. Results indicated a significant difference between the groups. The experimental group perceived less pain and demonstrated less behavioral distress than the control group did.

Another experimental study (Hansell et al., 1998), mentioned in chapter 2, was designed to measure stress, coping, and social support and to test the effect of a social support boosting intervention on levels of stress, coping, and social support among caregivers of children with HIV/AIDS. The sample was first stratified according to the caregivers' HIV status to ensure equal number of seropositive caregivers (biological parents) and seronegative caregivers (foster parents and extended family members) in each group. Caregivers were then randomly assigned to treatment groups. The two-group design compared participants who received monthly social support boosting intervention (experimental group) with those participants who did not receive the social support boosting intervention (control group). Levels of stress, coping, and social support were measured on entry into the study and at 6 months and 1 year. Statistically significant differences between the experimental and control groups were found in changes in the dependent variables over time when caregiver strata were included as a factor in the analysis; no statistically significant results were found when caregiver strata were combined. Univariate F tests indicated that the level of social support for caregivers who were seronegative in the experimental group was significantly different from seronegative caregivers in the control group and seropositive caregivers in both groups. No significant treatment group differences were found for seropositive caregivers. The researchers concluded that seronegative caregivers derived substantial benefit from the social support boosting intervention. Seronegative caregivers who acquire a child with HIV/AIDS are confronted with a complex stressful situation: the critical need to enhance their social support is achievable through the intervention tested in this study.

Not all experimental research follows the "true" experimental design. Campbell and Stanley (1963) have discussed six designs, three of which they called "pre-experimental," or sometimes "quasi-experimental" designs, and three "true" designs. The former usually do not include a control group or no randomization; while the latter provide for control groups and randomization. The pre-experimental design was used in a study by Elander and Hellstrom (1995) to see if a special educational program for nurses concerning causes of noise is effective in decreasing noise levels in an intensive care unit for infants. This design, in which nurses were tested before and after attending the program, is known as the one-group pretest-posttest design. For another example of a quantitative experimental design previously noted see Schepp (1991).

QUALITATIVE RESEARCH DESIGNS

Three common approaches used in qualitative research—phenomonology, ethnography, and grounded theory—were introduced in chapter 2. Phenomenology was described as a rigorous, critical, systematic investigation of a phenomenon central to the life experience of human beings about which little has been previously documented (Carpenter, 1995). An investigator may use ethnography to learn about a particular culture or situation by becoming a part of the culture or situation under investigation (Aamodt, 1991; Leininger, 1985). In grounded theory, which uses both an inductive and a deductive approach to theory development, data collection and analysis are concurrent and ongoing, with more specific data collected based on the analysis of initial data (Strauss & Corbin, 1994; Olshansky, 1996).

Increasingly, qualitative research in nursing is moving beyond simple production of specific baseline knowledge, nevertheless still greatly lacking in the discipline, to seek appropriate methods to examine the real meaning of these data (Byerly, 1987). Hermeneutics, a philosophy of science and a method of interpretation (Guba & Lincoln, 1989) has become a popular qualitative approach in the nursing research literature.

Hermeneutics is a phenomenological approach concerned with the description of an individual's experience and with the act of interpretation as a way to recover or point to the nature, or essence, of that experience. According to Chin (1986) hermeneutics acknowledges that human expressions contain a meaningful component that has to be recognized by subjects and transposed into their own system of values and meanings. Although the natural sciences are concerned with explanation and consider a theory of explanation necessary and sufficient for a theory of knowledge, hermeneuticists contend that something more is needed in a method to account for the intentionality and purposiveness of humans than mere explanation or description can offer. Herein lies the basis for the emphasis of hermeneutics on meaning and understanding (Chin, 1986, p. 139).

Rissmiller (1991) has made a significant contribution with her concise review, "Qualitative or Quantitative?" She comments, "It appears that nursing, in its quest for recognition as a science-based profession, is self-conscious about using a qualitative design, even though this approach may better suit the complex concepts and experiences appropriate for study by nurse researchers" (p. 1).

Smith (1998) noted that research in the area of problem drinking has traditionally relied on quantitative methodologies that view the problem from the researcher's perspective. The purpose of her hermeneutic study was to describe and understand the problem drinker's lived experience of suffering using a philosophy-and-research approach that preserves the uniqueness of the experience from the problem drinker's point of view. The method involved conducting in-depth interviews with a sample of six problem drinkers. Interviews were analyzed using an interpretive process that aimed at generating a deeper understanding of the topic by facilitating a fusion of the worldviews of both the participant and the researcher. The problem drinker's suffering was viewed as a spiraling vicious circle of physical, psychological, social, and spiritual distress. Symptoms of physical dependence, shame, and guilt emerged strongly as being both sequelae of heavy drinking and cues to further drinking bouts. Evoking memories of previous suffering through telling one's story was found to be an empowering and motivating force. Research methods such as the one used in this hermeneutic study encourage the voicing of individual experiences and emphasize understanding the meaning of experience from the individual's perspective.

Another example of how life experiences can be studied using a qualitative method is described by Feldman and Hott (1991). They showcase Trice's work (1991) on meaningful life experiences of older adults generating knowledge about health promotion and disease prevention in the elderly. Trice interviewed 2 men and 9 women, all White, from 65 to 87 years of age, who were living independently. He asked them "to describe any experience from life during which they had the sense their life was meaningful and had purpose" (p. 240). The overall themes that Trice gleaned from these very moving interviews suggests meaningfulness is perceived as doing something worthwhile, helpful, and needed and that this makes a difference in other people's lives. (It makes us wonder what a comparable qualitative study of nurse researchers would yield about meaningfulness in our lives!)

A phenomenological inquiry guided the research of Shaw (1997), who described the lived experience of the death of a peer during adolescence. According to Shaw, the limited literature dealing with the death of a peer did not include discussion from the perspective of the participant and focused on the immediate rather than the long-term aftermath of such an event. Therefore, understanding of the impact of adolescent loss was limited by the lack of rich and thorough individual description of the event and one's sense of the effect it had on subsequent psychosocial growth and development. This dearth of knowledge regarding this experience suggested a need for description and clarity best obtained through phenomenological inquiry. The detailed descriptions and reflections of the participants about their experience obtained through in-depth interviews was the primary source of data.

Schroeder (1996) selected a naturalistic, qualitative design for her study of womens' experience of bed rest in high-risk pregnancy because little substantive knowledge on this problem was available. Twelve adult pregnant women on prescribed bed rest of at least 3 weeks duration for a minimum of 20 hours per day were interviewed with the goal of understanding the experience of the participants as they themselves saw it. Interviews were allowed to flow from the directive, "Tell me about the experience of bed rest during your pregnancy." Three major themes that emerged from the data were the experience of high-risk pregnancy, the experience of bed rest, and the experience of time in high-risk pregnancy. Schroeder's work (1996) represents a beginning effort to contribute to nursing theory by her explanatory model of the experience of bed rest in high-risk pregnancy.

For another example of a well-done qualitative phenomenological study employing in-depth interviews, see Beck (1992). Compare it with her descriptive correlation design for her coauthored study (Beck, Reynolds, & Rutowski, 1992). It would be interesting to speculate how multimethod research using conceptual triangulation "to examine relationships among findings derived by different methods" (Foster, 1991, p. 44) would elaborate on Beck's research. Foster provides an integration model comprising five steps:

1. Developing criteria for inclusion of the findings in the model
2. Listing pertinent findings
3. Considering threats to the credibility of findings using paradigm-appropriate criteria
4. Examining relationships among the findings
5. Developing model(s) to represent the triangulated findings (1991, p. E44).

Knafl, Pettengill, Bevis, and Kirchhoff (1988) predicted a growing emphasis in nursing on combining quantitative and qualitative approaches in investigations. Morse (1991) provides an interesting discussion on various approaches to qualitative-quantitative methodological triangulation. Methodological triangulation is the use of at least two methods, usually qualitative and quantitative, to address the same research problem. Beck's research (1992) is an example of sequential triangulation, using a quantitative approach followed by qualitative approach. When a single research method is inadequate, triangulation helps to ensure that the most comprehensive approach is taken to solve a research problem.

The case study, although less often reported in nursing literature, is basically an in-depth survey that uses one subject. It is recognized as a suitable research tool for expanding our knowledge base and improving client services within nursing's domain. Although the case study method is most frequently used to report studies in psychiatric nursing, it can also be used in other clinical areas. For example, the special problems experienced by a mother who was breast-feeding preterm (34 weeks) quadruplets, reported by Mead, Chuffo, Lawlor-Klean, and Meier (1992) as a case study, provides research-based guidelines for clinicians to support breast-feeding in such situations. They found the case study method to be an ideal approach to studying this phenomenon, a problem of clinical significance that occurs infrequently. Based on the information from their intensive study of one mother, they concluded that mothers who want to breast-feed multiple newborns or infants should be supported in their decisions, and research-based interventions should be initiated as soon as possible after delivery. They encouraged nurses to report case studies on this topic so that practice can be guided by developing and expanding the general body of knowledge. Another interesting aspect of this case study is how it bears out the variables of achievement motivation and information noted by Rentschler (1991), in chapter 5. Graduate students may be gratified to know that Chuffo and Lawlor-Klean were in a nursing graduate program during one study and served as the primary care nurses during the neonates' hospitalization. This was a true case of hands-on research.

For another interesting example of a case study see. "One year in the life of a woman with premenstrual syndrome" (Lewis, 1995). The purpose of this study was to explore the subject of premenstrual syndrome (PMS) from the perspective of one woman's experience as she expressed it through daily Likert-scale symptom ratings and narrative journal entries for 1 year. For this subject, the findings provided evidence of predictive symptom patterns and an effect of symptom presence on her interpretation of her environment and herself.

THE HISTORICAL STUDY DESIGN

Although nurses have produced fewer historical studies than descriptive or experimental ones, interest in this type of inquiry is growing, particularly among doctoral candidates, who are increasingly basing their dissertations on historical research. The establishment of a National Nursing Archive within the Mugar Library was also an indication of this growing interest. This data bank of nursing history is an integral part of Boston University's Division of Special Collections. The Nursing Archive is made up of collections of personal and institutional papers, histories of schools of nursing, and early publications related to nursing. The Archive is the official depository of the ANA, the *American Journal of Nursing* company's historical collection, the Nursing Education Funds, Inc., materials, and materials from the AACN. The materials are maintained under optimal conditions, and the retrieval system makes them readily available to scholars.

In contrast to descriptive research, which is present oriented, and experimental research, which is predictive or future oriented, historical research is oriented to the past. Nevertheless, it is also a scientific search for truth and makes use of careful methods of collecting and analyzing data.

The purpose in doing a historical study will dictate the design for it. One cannot observe the events of the past nor set up an experiment to discover truths about past events. The major techniques used in historical research are documentation of the evidence and evaluation of its authenticity. These techniques stress the use of primary rather than secondary sources and involve both external and internal appraisal. In external appraisal the investigator asks, "How genuine is the material?" and "Is it what it purports to be?" In internal appraisal one asks, "How trustworthy is the material contained in the document?" Just as in descriptive research, historical research may start with a hunch or hypothesis, and it may produce hypotheses or generalizations. For example, you may say that the depression of the 1930s was a direct cause of the decline of private duty nursing in this country, that wars have always advanced the understanding of the need for nursing care, that the status and roles of women have had an influence on the advancement of nursing, and so forth.

Sources of information may include original manuscripts, official records, laws, letters, minutes of meetings, eyewitness accounts, newspaper accounts, diaries, biographies, memoirs, and oral histories on tapes or films. With the development and growing use of audiotape and videotape recorders, the preparation of oral and videotape histories has greatly increased as a means of recording history (Birnbach, 1985). All documents must be carefully evaluated for their authenticity, and primary sources must be distinguished from secondary sources. A primary source, published or unpublished, is one that gives direct evidence; for example, a letter that describes the philosophy or point of view of the letter writer is a primary source. A secondary source is a report that is one or more steps removed from the actual event described; if it is all you can find, you should look for several other secondary sources in order to verify the data to the extent possible. Even though you find corroborating evidence, however, your interpretations will have to remain guarded. The search for original materials may involve real detective work and be quite time consuming, but the experience of finding just the right material after much digging and searching is very satisfying.

The data found in a historical search must be evaluated for genuineness and relevance to the study in hand. It must be subjected to both external and internal criticism. External criticism involves asking whether the material is what it purports to be as to authorship, dates, and so forth. For example, was the letter you located really written by the person you are interested in? Sometimes letters are not dated, so the date will need to be established in some way. Or you may know to whom the letter was sent, but not the name of the sender. "Research into Things Past: Tracking Down One of Miss Nightingale's Correspondents" is an interesting account of methods used in tracing the recipient of a series of letters (Monteiro, 1972).

After the letter or other document has been authenticated, it may be subjected to internal criticism to determine the accuracy of the statements contained in it. Finally, the document must be examined for its relevance to the investigation. It may be an authentic primary source, but if it does not relate to your inquiry you cannot use it, no matter how interesting it is. Also, remember to examine the document in the context in which it was written or used. An understanding of the period in which it appeared is very important. Do not try to interpret or evaluate yesterday's documents by today's standards.

Historical research can be a most fascinating adventure. If you are interested in undertaking such a study, see Austin's (1958) classic article, "The Historical Method in Nursing." It contains suggestions and ideas about kinds of historical studies that might be undertaken as well as the author's own views on the subject. Historiography (Church, 1987) is rising, like the phoenix, to achieve full credibility and acceptance within the nursing profession. (Review chapter 2 for more on historical research.)

SUMMARY

In this chapter we have endeavored to show how one's research purpose helps in selecting a research design. We have discussed research methods and designs most commonly employed in quantitative nursing research: descriptive, longitudinal, cross-sectional, correlational, and experimental. Examples of various qualitative methods, the case study, and historical methods were also discussed. A variety of data collection methods used in research are presented in the next chapter, in which we also discuss the selection of a study sample.

REFERENCES

Aamodt, A. (1991). Ethnography and epistemology: Generating nursing knowledge. In J. Morse (Ed.), *Qualitative nursing research: A contemporary dialogue* (pp. 29–40). Newbury Park, CA: Sage.

Austin, A. L. (1958). The historical method in nursing. *Nursing Research, 7,* 4–10.

Beck, C. T. (1992). The lived experience of postpartum depression: A phenomenological study. *Nursing Research, 41,* 108–170.

Beck, C. T., Reynolds, M. A., & Rutowski, P. (1992). Maternity blues and postpartum depression. *Journal of Obstetric, Gynecologic, and Neonatal Nursing, 21,* 287–293.

Bergner, M., Bobbitt, R., Carter, W., & Gilson, B. (1981). The sickness impact profile: Development and final revision of a health status measure. *Medical Care, 19,* 787–805.

Birnbach, N. (1985). Recording Nursing's Past. The Oral History Project of the NYSNA. *Journal of the New York State Nurses Association, 16,* 7–9.

Byerly, E. L. (1987). Commentary. *Western Journal of Nursing Research, 9,* 239–241.

Campbell, D., & Stanley, J. (1963). *Experimental and quasi-experimental designs for research.* Chicago: Rand McNally.

Carpenter, D. (1995). Phenomenological research approach. In F. Steubert, & D. R. Carpenter (Eds.), *Qualitative research in nursing—advancing the humanistic imperative* (pp. 29–49). Philadelphia: J. B. Lippincott.

Chin, P. (1986). *Nursing research methodology,* Rockville, MD: Aspen Publications.

Church, O. (1987). Historiography in nursing research. *Western Journal of Nursing Research, 9,* 275–279.

Cusson, R., Madonia, J., & Taekman, J. (1997). The effect of environment on body site temperatures in full-term neonates. *Nursing Research, 46,* 202–207.

Elander, G., & Hellstrom, G. (1995). Reduction of noise levels in intensive car units for infants: Evaluation of an intervention program. *Heart and Lung, 24,* 376–379.

Fahs, P., & Kinney, M. (1991). The abdomen, thigh, and arm as sites for subcutaneous sodium heparin injections. *Nursing Research, 40,* 204–207.

Feldman, H. R., & Hott, J. R. (1991). Light up your practice with nursing research. *Journal of the New York State Nurses Association, 22,* 8–11.

Foster, R. (1991). A model to guide conceptual triangulation of quantitative and qualitative findings. 1991 International Nursing Research Conference. *Conference Abstracts, 44.*

Flo, G., & Brown, M. (1995). Comparing three methods of temperature taking: Oral mercury-in-glass, oral diatek, and tympanic first temp. *Nursing Research, 44,* 120–122.

Givin, B., Keilman, L., Collins, C., & Givin, W. (1990). Strategies to minimize attrition in longitudinal studies. *Nursing Research, 39,* 184–186.

Guba, E., & Lincoln, Y. (1989). *Fourth generation evaluation.* Newbury Park, CA: Sage.

Hansell, P., Hughes, C., Caliandro, G., Russo, P., Budin, W., Hartman, B., & Hernandez, O. (1998). The effects of a social support boosting intervention on stress, coping, and social support in caregivers of children with HIV/AIDS. *Nursing Research, 47,* 79–86.

Hoskins, C., Baker, S., Budin, W., Ekstrom, D., Maislin, G., Sherman, D., Steelman-Bohlander, J., Bookbinder, M., & Knauer, C. (1996a). Adjustment among husbands of women with breast cancer. *Journal of Psychosocial Oncology, 14*(1), 41–69.

Hoskins, C., Baker, S., Sherman, D., Bohlander, J., Bookbinder, M., Budin, W., Ekstrom, D., Knauer, C., & Maislin, G. (1996b). Social support and patterns of adjustment to breast cancer. *Scholarly Inquiry for Nursing Practice: An International Journal, 10*(2), 99–123.

Jackson, B., Taylor, J., & Pyngolil, M. (1991). How age conditions the relationship between climacteric status and health symptoms in African-American women. *Research in Nursing and Health, 14,* 1–9.

Knafl, K. A., Pettengill, M. M., Bevis, M. E., & Kirchhoff, K. T. (1988). Blending qualitative and quantitative approaches to instrument development and data collection. *Journal of Professional Nursing, 4,* 30–37.

Leininger, M. (1985). Ethnography and ethnonursing: Models and modes of qualitative data analysis. In M. Leininger (Ed.), *Qualitative research methods in nursing* (pp. 33–71). Orlando, FL: Grune & Stratton.

Lewis, L. (1995). One year in the life of a woman with premenstrual syndrome: A case study. *Nursing Research, 44,* 111–116.

Mason, D., & Redeker, N. (1993). Measurement of activity. *Nursing Research, 42,* 87–92.

Mason, D., & Tapp, W. (1992). Measuring circadian rhythms: Actigraph versus activation checklist. *Western Journal of Nursing Research, 14,* 358–379.

Mead, L. J., Chuffo, R., Lawlor-Klean, P., & Meier, P. P. (1992). Breastfeeding success in preterm quadruplets. *Journal of Obstetric, Gynecologic and Neonatal Nursing, 21,* 221–227.

Miller, K. M., & Perry, P. A. (1990). Relaxation technique and postoperational pain in patients undergoing cardiac surgery. *Heart & Lung, 19,* 136–146.

Monteiro, L. (1972). Research into things past: Tracking down one of Miss Nightingale's correspondents. *Nursing Research, 21,* 526–529.

Morse, J. (1991). Approaches to qualitative-quantitative methodological triangulation. *Nursing Research, 40,* 120–123.

Olshansky, E. (1996). Theoretical issues in building a grounded theory: application of an example of a program of research on infertility. *Qualitative Health Research, 6,* 394–405.

Porter, C., Oakley, D., Ronis, D., & Neal, W. (1996). Pathways of influence on fifth and eighth graders' reports about having had sexual intercourse. *Research in Nursing and Health, 19,* 193–204.

Redeker, N., Mason, D., Wykpisz, E., & Glica, B. (1996). Sleep patterns in women after coronary artery bypass surgery. *Applied Nursing Research, 9*(3), 115–122.

Rentschler, D. D. (1986). The relationship between pregnant women's achievement motivation, information about breastfeeding, and successful breastfeeding. *Dissertation Abstracts International, 47,* 4114B. (University Microfilms No. 8625–650).

Rentschler, D. D. (1991). Correlates of successful breastfeeding. *Image: Journal of Nursing Scholarship, 23,* 151–154.

Rissmiller, P. N. (1991). Qualitative or quantitative? *Nursing Scan in Research: Application for Clinical Practice, 4,* 1.

Salyer, J., Geddes, N., Smith, C., & Mark, B. (1998). *Nursing Research, 47,* 123–125.

Schepp, K. G. (1991). Factors influencing the coping efforts of mothers of hospitalized children. *Nursing Research, 40,* 42–46.

Schroeder, C. (1996). Women's experience of bed rest in high-risk pregnancy. *Image, 28,* 253–258.

Shaw, H. (1997). *Beyond grief: The extended impact of the death of a peer during adolescence among adult women. A phenomenological inquiry.* Unpublished doctoral dissertation. Adelphi University, Garden City, NY.

Smith, B. (1998). The problem drinker's lived experience of suffering: an exploration using hermeneutic phenomenology. *Journal of Advanced Nursing, 27*(1), 313–322.

Strauss, A., & Corbin, J. (1994). Grounded theory methodology. In N. Denzin, & Y. Lincoln (Eds.), *Handbook of qualitative research.* Thousand Oaks, CA: Sage.

Trice, L. B. (1991). Meaningful life experience in the elderly. *Image: Journal of Nursing Scholarship, 22,* 248–251.

Van Serellen, G., Lewis, C., & Leaka, B. (1990). The stresses of hospitalization among AIDS patients on integrated and special care units. *International Journal of Nursing Studies, 27,* 235–247.

Vessey, J., Carlson, K., & McGill, J. (1994). Use of distraction with children during an acute pain experience. *Nursing Research, 43,* 369–372.

Wong, D. & Baker, C. (1988). Pain in children: Comparison of assessment scales. *Pediatric Nursing, 14,* 9–17.

Yeaton, W., Smith, D., & Rogers, K. (1990). Evaluating understanding of popular press reports of health research. *Health Education Quarterly, 17,* 223–234.

Zeller, R., Good, M., Cranston-Anderson, G., & Zeller, D. (1997). Strengthening experimental design by balancing potentially confounding variables across treatment groups. *Nursing Research, 46,* 345–349.

7

Data Collection

After the investigator has defined the purpose, stated the hypothesis, and determined the design or method, the next logical steps involve choosing methods for collecting data and for selecting or developing a tool that will be used to collect the data. At the same time, thought must be given to the study population, commonly known as the sample.

METHODS OF COLLECTING DATA

Your reading of research reports in the nursing literature has undoubtedly made you aware of a variety of methods of collecting data. Research methods commonly used in nursing are observation, the interview, the questionnaire, rating scales, critical incidents, Q-sorts, the Delphi technique, diaries, record analyses, and nursing activity analyses. Quantitative research methods use a variety of these techniques. Qualitative approaches such as phenomenology, grounded theory, and ethnography use primarily observation and interviews. Sometimes approaches may overlap, because investigators use at least one and sometimes two or more of these methods of data collection.

For example, in studying perimenstrual symptoms and health-seeking behavior, Woods, Taylor, Mitchell, and Lentz (1992) used both a 90-day diary and an in-house interview. Following the completion of the diary, all women were asked to complete a telephone interview. The telephone interview may be, as Taussig and Freeman (1988) describe it, "the next best thing to being there." They suggest that telephone interviewing is a useful way to gather clinical information, reducing "lost to follow-up" numbers. In Woods et al. (1992), the sample of women who completed telephone interviews was not significantly different from the total sample with respect to demographic characteristics and so was representative of the clinical sample.

In a study designed to evaluate the validity and reliability of telephone interview data compared with the alternatives of in-person interviews and self-report questionnaires in an urban Spanish-speaking population, Lorig, Gonzalez, Ritter, and DeBrey (1997) found the quantity and quality of data collected by telephone were similar to what was collected by face-to-face interview. Although the quantity of data collected by questionnaire was significantly less than that collected by the other two methods, the quality of the data was the same. These authors concluded that data from Spanish-speaking subjects can be reliably collected using a telephone interview or mailed, self-administered Spanish-language questionnaires. In another study that examined response rates of posthospitalization telephone survey data, Minnick, Roberts, Young, Kleinpell, and Micek (1995) compared response-rate differences and reasons for nonparticipation by gender, age, ethnicity, and race. Race and gender did not relate to completion of the posthospitalization telephone interview. In fact, Whites and Blacks had virtually identical rates of completion. Younger patients, however, were slightly more likely to respond as compared with those more than 70 years old. Certainly, nurse researchers should be considering the telephone interview as one of a variety of ways to collect data or follow-up data, particularly after initial personal contacts have been made with participants.

Observation

Observation alone, or in combination with another method such as the interview or the questionnaire, is frequently used in nursing research. Observers may be concealed or unconcealed, or they may have characteristics of both these types. For example, the investigator may observe behavior through a two-way mirror while those observed are completely unaware of this presence. Of course, this kind of observation does not influence the behavior of the subjects, since they are unaware of the fact that they are being observed. This method raises ethical questions that the investigator must answer, however.

Most commonly, the observer is known to the subjects. This was the case in the exploratory study in which Engebretson (1996) wanted to observe and compare the models of healing and health used by nurses and alternative healers. Each nurse or healer to be observed was told why the observations were being made and was asked to participate. A major handicap that arises in this kind of observation is the influence of the observer on the observed; it is generally conceded that subjects tend to try to help the researcher by behaving as they believe the researcher wants them to. Does the mere participation in a study affect a subject's behavior and produce a "Hawthorne effect," in which respondents who know they are part of a research project alter their actions and behave in a way different from what is normal for them? The Hawthorne effect was named for studies conducted to find out the effects of various working conditions on worker productivity at the Hawthorne plant of the Western Electric Company. Investigators found that productivity increased regardless of what changes were made in work conditions. They concluded that the increased productivity was a result of the participants' knowledge that they were involved in a research study. Engebretson may have guarded against this behavior by explaining to both the nurses and the alternative healers that the reason they were being observed was to learn about the ways they heal and their concepts of health. It is unlikely that the participants were told that the observers would make comparisons between the nurses and the alternative healers, thus reducing the chance that the observer's presence would influence their responses.

A completely different type of observer, one who becomes a complete participant in the study, may or may not be recognized as an observer. For example, when nurses working on a unit are used as observers, they are accepted as a natural part of the environment and can collect data without the patients becoming aware that they are being observed. An example of participant observation was described by Killion (1995). She discussed this role of participant observer in relation to an ethnographic study of homeless pregnant women in Southern California. In a study such as this, the investigator becomes a part of the situation under investigation. For example, Killion spent time with the women in the shelters and accompanied them to the emergency department, housing authority, welfare office, and health clinics and while grocery shopping, and apartment and job hunting. The intense social interaction with the women in their own milieu allowed the researcher to witness the homeless experience through the eyes of the women. In another qualitative study, Schroeder (1996) used both observation and interview techniques to obtain data on the experience of bed rest in high risk pregnancy. Data sources included medical records, demographic information, field notes documenting the researcher's experiences as participant-observer, audiotapes of interviews, and computer transcripts of the taped interview. Using these data, she categorized her findings under three major themes: perceptions of high-risk pregnancy, perceptions of bed rest, and the experience of time and restricted movement. Schroeder (1996) concluded with an interesting discussion of nursing implications to be derived from her study. Her final conclusion was that this routine obstetric intervention (bed rest) should be seriously evaluated in light of its lack of demonstrated effectiveness and because it has potential for seriously harming women and their families.

Another qualitative approach to data collection is the grounded theory method. In this technique, data collection and analysis are concurrent and ongoing, with more specific data collected based on the analysis of initial data. Olshansky has written extensively on the use and process of grounded theory and employed it in her studies of women's infertility (see Olshansky, 1987, 1990, 1996; Woods, Olshansky, & Draye, 1991). In her 1996 article, Olshansky presents an outstanding example of a program of research on infertility whereby a grounded theory of identity of self as an infertile person was developed and elaborated on. She also raises theoretical questions about grounded theory methodology in an effort to advance our thinking about this methodology and how it can contribute to theory generation through linked studies in a program of research. Wagnild and Young (1990) also used a grounded theory approach, identifying five underlying themes that were thought to constitute resilience in older women: equanimity, self-reliance, existential aloneness, perseverance, and meaningfulness.

Unlike using qualitative approaches in which the participant observer allows the meaning of the experience to unfold, when using quantitative approaches, the participant observer often encounters difficulty while trying to maintain objectivity. Participant observers may find it helpful to use a tool designed to guide the observations or to record observations, thus helping to provide uniform data. Whether the data are collected by one observer or more than one, the type of data collected on each observation should be the same. Furthermore, observers need training in the use of the observation tool to strengthen the reliability of the observations, that is, to ensure that the observers are using the same approach to collection of the data and that they maintain this reliability throughout the period of data collection. Mariano (1990) suggests a creative exercise to learn the skill needed for observational data collection. In one, described as "a miniparticipant-observation exercise" (p. 356), you spend approximately 1 hour in a public place unfamiliar to you—a supermarket, playground, or bus or train station—where you assume the role of a field researcher, observing the setting, atmosphere, people, and interactions. Immediately after, write as detailed and comprehensive notes as you can, including your own feelings about the experience, and a short analysis of your observations, abstracting one or two themes suggested by the data. These observation notes are then brought to class for discussion and critique. This docs not have to be confined to a class, however. A research study group could find this a productive, imaginative way to discuss observation as part of the research process.

The Interview

In studies in which the investigator is interested in obtaining facts, ideas, impressions, or opinions from the study subjects, and when it is possible for you or your assistants to be in personal contact with the study subjects, you may elect to use the interview method of data collection.

Interviews are of two types: structured and unstructured. The type used will depend on the researcher's purpose in using the interview method of gathering data. For example, in a qualitative study, the interview is usually unstructured. The structured interview is somewhat akin to the questionnaire in that each interview follows a set pattern of questioning, with the wording and sequencing of questions the same for all respondents (Hutchinson & Wilson, 1992).

In the study by Van Servellen, Lewis, and Leake (1990) to assess how the number and perception of stressors associated with hospitalization for AIDS could be reduced, the researchers used a structured face-to-face interview in which each patient was asked to indicate (a) whether a particular item applicable to the complication of AIDS was a stressor and (b) the extent to which the AIDS patient was bothered by it. Analysis of the 370 interviews (280 from special care units and 90 from integrated units) slightly favored the special care unit. It is important here to note that the structured questions had been especially adapted for AIDS patients from a hospital stress rating scale (Volicer & Bohannon, 1975), raising questions about whether the validity and reliability of the revised instrument had been established.

The structured interview can be more objectively and easily tabulated than an unstructured interview can be. Questions used must be carefully chosen to obtain the data needed, however. As mentioned earlier, the questions asked in interviews are similar to those included in questionnaires, but the data are collected in person, allowing for some probing when the answers to questions are not clearly understood at first.

Another example of in-depth structured interviews is seen in Beck's (1992) phenomenological study of the essential structure of the lived experience of postpartum depression as described by a purposive sample of seven mothers who had attended a local postpartum depression support group that Beck had helped to facilitate. She structured the interview by asking participants to respond the following statement: "Please describe a situation in which you experienced postpartum depression. Share all the thoughts, perceptions, and feelings you can recall until you have no more to say about the situation."

A scheduled semistructured interview requires all respondents to give certain types of information but permits some flexibility in phrasing and the order of the questions stemming from the respondents' characteristics (Hutchinson & Wilson, 1992). Huchinson and Wilson (1992) draw an illuminating map of how to avoid the kinds of validity threats to interview techniques that manifest themselves, even for the most experienced interviewer. They point out the penalty, as well as the reward, of using interviews in producing credible research. Carpenter (1998) described benefits spontaneously reported by women who participated in a descriptive study of self-esteem and well-being. Many women described participating in terms of a therapeutic intervention that deeply affected them. Women described the research as an opportunity to review their thoughts and feelings about both themselves and their lives with an active listener. Unanticipated benefits of participating in research interviews reported by Hutchinson, Wilson, and Wilson (1994) included catharsis, self-acknowledgment, sense of purpose, self-awareness, empowerment, healing, and providing a voice for the disenfranchised.

The data obtained in the less formalized unstructured interview, which uses the open-end type of question in order to obtain freer responses, are more difficult to analyze than those obtained in a structured interview are. In unstructured interviews the content must be analyzed according to pre-established identification of the categories. Content analysis requires categorizations and judgments of responses made by expert judges who are usually not the interviewers. This kind of planning and use of judges helps to ensure the validity and reliability of the content analysis. Brennan, Moore, and Smyth (1995) used content analysis in a study of the effects of a special computer network on caregivers of persons with Alzheimer's. In this study, the caregiver could access a computer network that was specially designed to provide information, communication, and decision-support functions for caregivers of persons with Alzheimer's disease. The unstructured messages posted on the computer network provided data similar to those obtained in an unstructured interview. Using content analysis, the 622 messages posted by the caregivers were organized according to seven predetermined categorizations designed by Toseland and Rossiter (1989) in their review of themes present in support groups for caregivers of older persons with dementia. The frequency of these themes reported in the posted messages was as follows:

> Group and its members as a mutual support group system (37%); Information about the care recipient's situation (24%); Emotional impact of caregiving (19%); Development and use of support systems outside the group (13%); Problematic interpersonal relationships (4%); Self-care (3%); and Home-care skills (2%). (Toseland & Rossiter, 1989, p. 170)

Lothian (1995) describes the complex process involved in the analysis of the rich contextual data obtained in her qualitative study that explored the baby's role in successful breast-feeding. In this study data collection and analysis were concurrent. Extensive field notes were developed, coded, and analyzed. As codes were developed and categories emerged, hypotheses were developed and tested during the next visits. The families were compared with each other, and eventually the literature was reviewed as another comparison group.

The Questionnaire

The questionnaire (or "opinionnaire") is a paper-and-pencil approach to the collection of quantitative data. Its advantage over the interview is that it can be used with subjects at a distance without greatly increasing the cost and time involved. It is most useful in surveys of large groups of people. The U.S. government's population census is a good example of the use of the questionnaire to survey a large number of people over a wide area.

Questionnaires may be employed to obtain demographic data, that is, social or vital statistics such as age, sex, marital status, educational background, and so forth. They can also be used to obtain information about certain types of phenomena; for example, Garrett (1991) gathered data about the leadership preferences, head nurse leader style, and job satisfaction of staff nurses by means of a mailed questionnaire survey to a proportional random sample of 198 direct caregiver RNs selected from three federal tertiary care facilities in different regions of New York State. The demographic data Garrett collected from 188 RNs (62% response rate) indicated that the nurses in the sample were generally representative of the Veterans' Administration system nationwide, of New York State, and of the nation. The demographic data collected by the questionnaire thus not only described her sample but also provided a comparison with other nursing populations. Keane (1991) is another investigator who used a questionnaire to study nurses' attitudes, in this case, the effects of a psychiatric nursing curriculum on an ethnically and linguistically diverse nursing student population. The questionnaire Opinions about Mental Illness (Cohen & Struening, 1963) plus additional items by Link, McNamara, Penney, and Ungemack (1978) were given to four classes of upper junior baccalaureate students prior to their senior-level psychiatric nursing course (experimental group). At the same time upper sophomore nursing students who were in a medical-surgical nursing course became a convenience sample (control group). Pretest questionnaires were given out and completed in class and then distributed to each group 6 months later when the experimental group had completed their psychiatric nursing course (posttest).

Keane (1991) found that new knowledge about mental illness and direct contact with psychiatric patients did contribute to attitude change in four out of five dimensions in this culturally diverse student nurse sample. The five dimensions were authoritarianism; social restrictiveness; community residence; welcome home, a perception that the mentally ill integrate into communities better with support services; and stereotyping. The attitude that didn't change was stereotyping. Keane concludes that more information relative to stereotyping (and authoritarianism) needs to be explored in academic and clinical nursing content. Isn't nursing research challenging?

In addition to descriptive data about phenomena such as those collected by Garrett (1991) and Keane (1991), information about perceptions and attitudes can also be sought by questionnaire. In the Budin (1998) study, participants completed a four-part questionnaire that included (a) the Psychosocial Adjustment to Breast Cancer Factor Score (Murphy, 1994) of the Psychosocial Adjustment to Illness Scale (PAIS) (Derogatis, 1983); (b) the Symptom Distress Scale (SDS) (McCorkle & Young, 1978); (c) the Social Support Network Inventory (SSNI) (Flaherty, Gaviria, & Pathak, 1983); and (d) a demographic information form. These instruments, which measured perceptions of adjustment, symptom distress, and social support, were all used in previous research and had well-established reliability and validity. Making use of suitable, valid, and reliable tools already available not only saves time but also enables one to make comparisons of one's findings with the results of others also using these tools.

The questions in a questionnaire can be either closed, for example, true–false or answerable by "yes" or "no," or open-ended. Answers obtained by open-ended questions, such as those obtained by unstructured interviews, are somewhat more difficult to analyze than are those obtained by closed questions. Some questionnaires contain both closed and open-ended questions, the latter being included for the purpose of obtaining a freer response. The purpose in using the questionnaire will help the investigator select the type of questions to use.

Success in using the questionnaire depends on how carefully it is constructed. First, the questions should cover the significant area to be studied. Thus, a good questionnaire is based on previous study. Either the questions have already been tested in previous research, as they were in the Budin study, or they are based on careful observation, experience, consultation with experts, and systematic review of the literature. Review the questions raised in the Van Servellen et al. (1990) variation of the Volicer and Bohannon (1975) questionnaire for AIDS patients. Second, the questions should be worded as carefully as possible to ensure understanding. There are many excellent references that provide information about phrasing questions in questionnaires (see Burns & Grove, 1997; Polit & Hungler, 1995; Waltz, Strickland, & Lenz, 1991). Third, the questions should be pretested on a group that is similar to but not the same as the sample you plan to study. The importance of this pretesting cannot be overemphasized. It should always be done unless the questions you plan to use have already been successfully tested in previous research and found to be valid and reliable.

One of the limitations of the questionnaire is the fact that not all individuals in the sample you select will return the questionnaire, and some of those who do return it will not answer all the questions, making their responses useless. Another limitation lies in the difficulty of constructing questions that will be interpreted in the same way by all the respondents. Furthermore, there may be a tendency on the part of the respondents to give answers they think are wanted. This "Hawthorne effect," in which individuals behave or respond differently than the way they normally would because they know they are participating in a research study, has been mentioned earlier. Keeping the respondent anonymous by asking respondents not to sign the questionnaire will help avoid this latter problem to some extent. Of course, questionnaires should always be accompanied by a stamped, self-addressed return envelope.

For an excellent article on improving response rate to mailed questionnaires, see Gordon and Stokes (1989). These authors noted that the mailed questionnaire is an important data collection method in research because of the ease with which large samples can be reached at relatively low cost in comparison with face-to-face data collection methods. They acknowledged, however, that the mailed questionnaire often has a reduced response rate, which casts serious doubt on the representative nature of the sample. To help improve response rates these authors provided a number of helpful suggestions, including a variety of personal touches to make the participants feel committed, valued, and appreciated, such as personalized letters emphasizing the importance of the study and thanking individuals for participating. These methods are aimed at helping participants develop a commitment to the study. The credibility of the study is also enhanced by using university or hospital letterhead and return address. Mechanical strategies aimed at enhancing the ease of response include the use of attractive, easy-to-use questionnaires; color coding; self-addressed, stamped envelopes; and follow-up reminders.

Costs associated with a direct mail survey were addressed in a marketing research study funded by the New York Counties Registered Nurses Association (Camuñas, Alward, & Vecchione, 1990). Their 22-item questionnaire was sent to a random sample of 70 RNs, members of the NYSNA. Their response rate was directly attributable to the technique employed. When they used a monetary incentive ($1.00) the response rate increased significantly; when they provided information about the association, response rates decreased significantly. When they combined a direct mailing to complete questionnaires and to solicit for more membership, neither technique was effective. In this study, money talked.

Rating Scales

Rating scales are useful when one is trying to obtain a numerical or verbal value judgment of some element, factor, or program, such as a measurement of satisfaction with nursing care. Rating scales may also be used to obtain subjective responses about attitudes, personal ideas, or impressions. For example, in the study that investigated the relationships among spirituality, perceived social support, death anxiety, and nurses' willingness to care for AIDS patients, Sherman (1996) used a variety of standardized instruments to measure these concepts. For example, the Templer Death Anxiety Scale (Templer, 1970), one of the most widely used measures of conscious death anxiety, consists of 15 true or false items, with scores ranging from 0 to 15. Higher scores indicate higher death anxiety. Some of the problems attending the use of a rating scale to determine attitudes toward death are discussed. Perceived social support was measured by the Personal Resource Questionnaire-85 (Brandt & Weinert, 1987). This instrument consists of 25 items with a Likert seven-point response format. A Likert scale is a type of composite measure of attitudes that involves summation of scores on a set of items to which respondents are asked to indicate their degree of agreement or disagreement. The above study (Brandt & Weinert, 1987) used a 7-point scale. Most rating scales are set up as either 3- or 5-point scales. A broader scale may be used, but there may be a tendency for respondents to avoid the extremes that occur when the scale is broad. Rating scales may be set up as equal-interval scales and numerical values given to the intervals. They may also be set up to rate qualitative or ordinal data, using some criteria such as "least valuable, moderately valuable, most valuable." Flaskerud (1988) questioned whether the Likert scale format was culturally biased. She speculated that problems in using Likert scales cross-culturally could be due to education, faulty translation, irrelevant content, lack of semantic equivalence, the differing character of social interactions in various groups, or the nature of the response required. It is also possible that the degree of variation Likert scales attempt to measure is meaningless to some cultural groups. This thoughtful article raises the question so other investigators may become aware of potential difficulties when choosing or developing an instrument.

Another tool often used to measure subjective experiences such as pain, nausea, fatigue, and dyspnea is the VAS (Gift, 1989). This self-report device consists of a line, usually 100 mm in length, with anchors at each end to indicate the extremes of the sensation under study. The subject is asked to mark a point that indicates the amount of the sensation experienced at the time. The intensity of the sensation is scored by measuring the millimeters from the low end of the scale to the subject's mark. When used properly, the VAS is an easy-to-use, reliable, valid, and sensitive self-report measure for studying subjective patient experiences (Fig. 7.1).

A rating scale that is especially useful for children is the Wong-Baker Faces Pain Rating Scale (Wong & Baker, 1988). This instrument consists of a series of six faces that range from very happy to very sad and tearful, placed horizontally on a piece of paper (Fig. 7.2).

The individual administering the rating scale explains to the child that each face is for a person who feels happy because he has no pain (hurt) or sad because he has some or a lot of pain. Face 0 is very happy because he doesn't hurt at all. Face 1 hurts just a little bit. Face 2 hurts a little more. Face 3 hurts even more. Face 4 hurts a whole lot. Face 5 hurts as much as you can imagine, although you don't have to be crying to feel this bad. The examiner then asks the child to choose the face that best describes how he or she is feeling. This instrument is scored as a Likert scale, with scores ranging from 0 (very happy) to 5 (tearful). Wong and Baker reported excellent reliability and validity of this instrument for children 3 to 18 years of age. Vessey, Carlson, and McGill (1994) used this instrument as a measure of pain in their experimental study of the use of distraction with children during an acute pain experience (see chapter 6).

The Critical Incident Technique

The critical incident technique for obtaining data involves the use of written reports that describe previous experiences or observations. Von Post (1996) explored ethical dilemmas in perioperative nursing practice through the use of the critical incident technique. The aim of the study was to elicit the ethical dilemmas that arise in perioperative nurses' practice. An analysis of the critical incidents identified four domains of ethical dilemmas: those arising as value conflicts in the intraoperative phase of surgery, those emanating from the patient's right of

No pain at all /--/ Pain as bad as it could be

FIGURE 7.1 Visual Analog Scale (VAS).

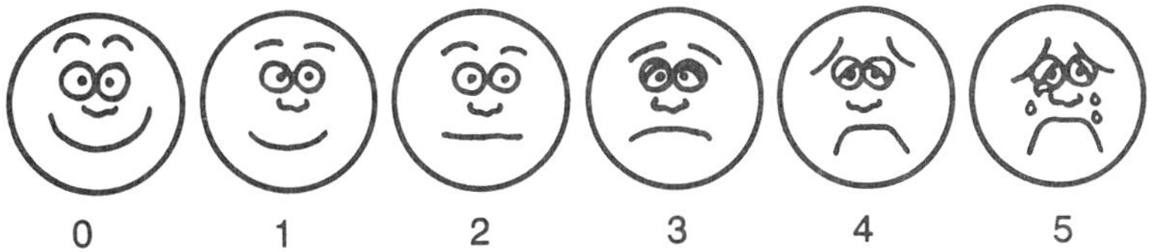

FIGURE 7.2 Wong-Baker Faces Pain Rating Scale.

Note: From *Wong and Whaley's Clinical Manual of Pediatric Nursing* (4th ed., p. 316) by D. L. Wong, 1996, St. Louis, MO: C. V. Mosby. Copyright 1996 by C. V. Mosby. Reprinted with permission.

self-determination, those arising in caring for patients, and those resulting from the allocation of scarce resources and the demands of increased effectiveness. Critical incident reports are based on the subject's memory of incidents that involved human activities. The activity described must be sufficiently complete in itself to illustrate the behavior under study. The incident as written by the subject is analyzed in terms of content categories developed by the investigator. Again, categorization of the material is more objective when done by independent expert judges other than the investigator.

The Q-Sort Technique

The Q-sort technique has been used at times in nursing research. This technique consists of a set of cards on each of which a statement is printed. The subject is asked to sort the cards into a specified number of piles according to the importance of the statement. In an interesting study, von Essen and Sjoden (1993) identified psychiatric inpatient and staff perceptions of most and least important nurse caring behaviors using a modified Swedish version of the CARE-Q instrument. The CARE-Q is based on Q-sort methodology. It consists of 50 caring behaviors that are to be placed along a continuum of significance, and the subject is instructed to rank them in seven categories from most important to least important. The final distribution is required to conform to a symmetrical, quasi-normal distribution (see chapter 8) by asking the individuals to identify 1 most and 1 least important item, 4 next most and 4 next least important items, 10 rather and 10 not so important items, and 20 items that are neither important nor unimportant. Each behavior was given a value from 1 to 7 according to the individual's placement of it in a category. Mean values and mean rankings are then calculated for each item.

The Q-sort is usually a difficult task for the subject. The job can be made easier, however, if directions are carefully given and if the subject understands the importance of the study. For another example of a study that used Q-sort, see Wingate and Lackey (1989). To identify the needs of the noninstitutionalized patient with cancer as defined by patients, primary caregivers, and nurses and to identify the needs of the primary caregiver as defined by the same three groups of subjects, each subject completed two forms of an open-ended questionnaire on which they were asked to list the needs of patients and caregivers. From these lists they applied content analysis to the two data sets to arrive at categories of need responses. Then each set of data, with category labels and definitions, underwent a Q-sort technique by two successive groups of nurse experts to establish the validity of the need item responses in categories. The Q-sort results showed the psychological needs category with the largest number of needs for both patients and caregivers. The physical and information needs was the next largest for patients and household management (patient care) and information needs were second and third largest for caregivers.

The Delphi Technique

The Delphi technique or procedure is a special type of survey developed at the Rand Corporation (Pill, 1970) It is a device for tapping the ideas of a knowledgeable group of people by mail survey. It consists of a series of rounds of questioning using a panel of experts or persons representing the field under study. The purpose is usually to arrive at consensus of opinion on some important subject for the purpose of predicting the future, for developing program planning, or for project evaluation.

The procedure includes the following steps:

- Development of a representative panel that consents to participate in the survey. The panel members are contacted personally or by mail to explain the survey and to solicit their participation.
- Round one solicits the opinions of the panel members on the subject under study. Usually they are requested to list a specified number of ideas or opinions. These opinions are then combined and returned to the panel members, who are asked to select a specified number of the most important ones. In the remaining rounds, the opinions are further limited to those that survive the consensus of the group.

The Delphi technique provides a simple way of obtaining the opinions of a large group of experts and of obtaining consensus among them without the problems inherent in a face-to-face meeting, where consensus may mean acceptance of the ideas of the most vocal or prestigious group members. Thus, the technique preserves anonymity, provides controlled feedback, and promotes group consensus. It may, of course, tend toward some lack of truly creative ideas or predictions, since consensus tends to move a group toward the more conservative opinions. Abdellah and Levine (1986) consider Delphi data to be subjective and judgmental.

Forte, Ritz, and Balestracci (1997) used a Delphi technique for identifying nursing research priorities in a newly merged health care system. Using a 110-member panel, the study identified two final topics that were focused on nursing administration research. Collecting these data served many purposes, including increased organizational awareness about nursing research and development of a nursing research council to facilitate future activities.

To identify competencies needed by nurse leaders in public health programs, a five-round national Delphi survey was carried out (Misener et al., 1997) using a convenience sample of members of major public health nursing associations and nurse and nonnurse public health leaders in the United States. Initially, 62 competencies were identified. Factor analysis resulted in four factors: political competencies, business acumen, program leadership, and management capabilities. These researchers concluded that graduate schools in nursing and public health must prepare students with broad-based competencies from a variety of disciplines. Findings from this national survey provided a database for curriculum development and evaluation of programs to prepare nurse leaders for roles in public health–based delivery systems.

The Delphi technique was also used by a nursing research committee at a large tertiary care teaching hospital (Nappier, Stanfield, Simon, Bennett, & Gowan, 1990) to identify clinical nursing research priorities so that nursing research in clinical practice could be facilitated. This technique was chosen as their first research venture because of its simplicity and the shared individual and collective responsibility of all committee members. It promoted collaboration between the research committee members as data collectors and required essential input and participation of staff nurses in clinical practice, nurse administrators, and educators. The nurses identified 74 research questions for their potential impact on patients. The top priority rankings were nursing recruitment and retention, discharge planning, primary nursing, patient education, patient satisfaction, QA, patient outcomes, and specific nursing interventions. These priorities opened the block that had inhibited nursing research at this institution. (For excellent references on this technique see Crisp, Pelletier, Duffield, Adams, & Nagy, 1997; Schmidt et al., 1997; and Williams & Webb, 1994).

Other Techniques and Tools

In addition to the major data collection techniques we have been discussing, several other techniques are available. Existing records such as nurses' notes, Kardexes, and medical records are commonly used in both ongoing and retrospective research. Micelli, Waxman, Cavalieri, and Lage (1994) used nursing assessment records, medical records, physician progress notes, and order sheets to examine falls among older nursing home residents. A retrospective chart review of all the nurse-patient clinic encounters for a 6-month period provided data for Skrutkowska and Weijer (1997) to examine differences in nursing care received by patients with breast cancer enrolled in clinical trials and those not enrolled in clinical trials. Iglesias (1998) used existing records in a retrospective descriptive study designed to analyze the current specialty practice of the community mental health clinical nurse specialist (CNS) and to identify possible areas for expansion of mental health nursing services offered at home by a visiting nurse agency. The data for this study were collected by the investigator from patient charts and CNS referral forms at a large home health care agency. The author explains that when a referring nurse requests a CNS psychosocial assessment, a CNS referral form is completed, including basic demographic and scheduling information, current nursing interventions, and assessment concerns. The CNS documentation on the referral forms and the patient charts were analyzed to provide evidence to support the need for role expansion of the mental health CNS in home care.

The use of existing records presents problems, however, since errors and omissions occur in recording, as is well known (Aaronson & Burman, 1994). Some of these errors can be overcome in ongoing research by careful preparation of the nurses doing the recording. In retrospective or historical research, no control can be exercised, and the investigator must use what is there and verify it in other ways, such as by comparison with other contemporary records.

A health diary is a useful methodological tool used in both research and clinical practice to examine the daily symptoms of healthy and ill people, responses to symptoms, and efficacy of symptom response. Health diaries have been used with a variety of patient populations, including children (Butz & Alexander, 1991), women with menstrual problems (Heitkemper, Jarrett, Bond, & Turner, 1991; Seideman, 1990; Woods et al., 1992), and individuals with cancer (Oleske, Heinze, & Otte, 1990). Diaries are usually constructed using one of two general formats: as a journal in which health events are all entered on the same page for each day like a calendar or in a ledger in which separate pages are used for different types of events. The use of diaries to examine day-to-day problems can result in high data quality. For an excellent overview of health diaries in nursing research and practice, see Burman (1995).

A data collection technique that has been used in nursing studies for a number of years is the nursing activity analysis. This technique has been considered more helpful in problem solving than in actual research. The purpose of studies using this method is to determine how nursing personnel spend their time, and particularly how this time is divided between patient care and other unit activities.

Although tools used to record observations are often of the checklist variety, other possible tools are printouts of monitoring systems, fieldwork notes, and videotapes. Fieldwork notes are often used by anthropologists when studying the culture of groups of people. This special kind of recording focuses on the investigator's specific area of interest. Videotapes can provide an efficient and reliable record for analysis of behaviors. Recent developments in lightweight, technologically advanced video cameras have overcome many of the obstacles associated with visual recordings in the past. Videotapes offer efficiency in the data collection process because they record rich and permanent documentation of behaviors. At the same time, researchers are cautioned to take into consideration factors such as cost, possible Hawthorne effect, and issues concerning informed consent and privacy. For excellent articles on the use of videotapes in research see Roberts, Srour, and Winkelman (1996) and Heacock, Souder, and Chastain (1996).

Locating Data Collection Instruments

A glance through the nursing research and specialty journals that dedicate more than 50% of the publication to research in practice, education, or administration will give you some indication of the many diverse tools used in quantitative research. Some are used to collect data, others to record data that have been collected. Some of those are checklists, such as Duffy's (1985) Research Appraisal Checklist (RAC) 6-point Likert scale with 51 criteria that Brown (1990) used to appraise research reports of diabetes patient research (see chapter 3). In the *Journal of Neuroscience Nursing,* Hilton, Sisson, and Freeman (1990) reported on piloting the use of a Neurobehavioral Rating Scale (NRS) that has been used for rapid bedside assessment of patients with closed head injuries and stroke to evaluate and aid in monitoring neurological deterioration. It was also used to assist in appropriate placement of patients with AIDS and dementia complex and to plan their care. The NRS, a 7-point Likert scale of 27 items, was tested to evaluate its interrater reliability in determining emotional and behavioral responses in the seropositive HIV population. Although the small sample ($N = 9$) must be taken into consideration, the tool appears useful.

An interesting tool used for predicting pressure sore risk used in a variety of studies dealing with decubitus ulcers is the Braden Scale (Day, Hayes, Kennedy, & Diercksen, 1997). This scale is composed of six subscales that reflect sensory perception, skin moisture, activity, mobility, friction, and shear and nutritional status. This instrument has highly satisfactory reliability when used by RNs and greater sensitivity and specificity than do instruments previously reported. In a comparison study of risk assessment tools currently in use, Goodridge (1993) found the Braden Scale to be the only tool that demonstrates good reliability ratings (0.89 to 0.99).

After reviewing reports in nursing research journals, you may find that several different instruments have been used to evaluate similar topics (Kemp, 1990). For example, the Beck Depression Inventory and the Stein Maternity Blues Scale were used by Beck, Reynolds, and Rutowski (1992) in one descriptive correlational study and in-depth interviews were used in a qualitative study to describe the essential nature of the lived experience of postpartum depression (Beck, 1992). Jones and Kay (1992) point out the problems in developing instruments for cross-cultural research, such as developing instruments in a target language and matching translation strategy to the goals of the study (p. 186). A variety of tools and methods used to measure biophysiological variables, such as heart rate, blood pressure, temperature, muscle strength, nutrition, pulmonary artery pressure, cardiac output, oxygen saturation, blood glucose, and other laboratory reports, have been described in the nursing literature (Pugh & DeKeyser, 1995).

There are numerous resources for locating instruments. An excellent resource is *The Journal of Nursing Measurement* (Strickland, Hinshaw, & DiLorio, 1998). As the only journal that specifically addresses instrumentation in nursing, it serves as a forum for disseminating information on instruments, tools, approaches, and procedures developed or used for measuring variables in nursing. Waltz and Strickland have edited a multivolume set on measurements of nursing outcomes (1988a, 1988b, 1990, 1991). For another comprehensive listing and description of *Instruments for Clinical Health-Care Research* see Frank-Stromborg and Olsen (1997). Fitzpatrick's *Encyclopedia of Nursing Research* (1998) is the first book of its kind to provide comprehensive explanations of nursing research topics and services and affords extensive cross-references to assist in finding information, including measurements and scales. *The Health and Psychological Instruments Online* (HaPI), a computerized reference, is available in most university libraries. This computerized service provides information on questionnaires, rating scales, interview forms, checklists, vignettes or scenarios, indexes, coding schemes or manuals, projective techniques, and tests. Information is abstracted from leading journals covering the health and psychosocial sciences. Also covered are instruments from organizational behavior and library and information science beginning in 1985, with selective retrospective coverage.

Another excellent source for locating instruments is the Buros Institute of Mental Measurements. Buros (1998), which now can be accessed through the Internet, has a 50-year history of serving the public interest and advancing the field of measurement. By providing professional assistance, expertise, and information to users of commercially published tests, the Institute promotes meaningful and appropriate test selection, use, and practice. The Buros Institute encourages improved test development and measurement research through thoughtful, critical analysis of measurement instruments and the promotion of an open dialogue regarding contemporary measurement issues (Buros, 1998). The Institute's goals of serving the public interest and contributing positively to the measurement field are accomplished through several avenues: publication of the *Mental Measurements Yearbook* and *Tests in Print* series, presentation of the Buros-Nebraska Symposium on Measurement and Testing, sponsorship of the journal *Applied Measurement in Education,* and direct professional consultation.

A search using databases such as CINAHL or MEDLINE is also useful in locating information about a particular instrument you are interested in or for locating instruments that have been used for measuring specific concepts (this will be further developed in chapter 10). *Dissertation Abstracts* might also be useful in locating instruments that have never been published.

Snyder (1989), reviewing valid, reliable, and usable measurements, makes the salient point that establishing validity and reliability of an instrument, such as an inventory for measuring pain, requires time and expertise, so why reinvent the wheel? Nurses may find, however, that the population we wish to study is unique, such as AIDS patients, or a new phenomenon is being explored, as we noted earlier in Hilton et al. (1990). As in that study, instruments may need to be adapted or new ones developed (Snyder, 1989).

We have touched on only a few of the tools used to collect and record data in current use. You may be able to locate others in the research literature or even think of some yourself. Whatever method is used to collect and record data, it should be so constructed that different persons using the same tool will obtain the same kind of data. Observer reliability checks and the use of independent judges are two ways of ensuring this. In addition, in experimental studies you must make sure that the observers do not know which subjects are the controls and which are in the experimental group.

VALIDITY AND RELIABILITY OF DATA-COLLECTING INSTRUMENTS

In the foregoing discussion of methods of collecting and recording data, the words validity and reliability were used frequently because an evaluation of research findings requires that the validity and reliability of the tool be established.

The validity of a research tool refers to its ability to obtain the needed data. It tells the investigator whether the tool will measure what you want to measure. The term *face validity* is sometimes used to indicate that validity has been established simply by looking at a tool, a questionnaire or checklist, for example, or by having experts look at it to see whether the items are the important ones. This method of testing validity is the weakest one available.

A better way to test the measuring ability of a tool is to establish its *content validity*, which involves evaluating whether the questions on the instrument are representative of questions that should be asked about that topic (Kemp, 1990). To do this, the investigator points out the authority for the use of the content in the questions, checklist, or other type of tool. This authority may be derived from the literature, the investigator's personal observations, or consultation with others who are experts.

A still better, but more complex, method of testing validity involves testing results on the instrument with results from the use of another known instrument that tests the same sort of content. For example, if you are using a new tool to test for evidence of anxiety and you can find in the literature a valid test of anxiety that used another tool, you can then give both tests to a group and compare the results.

The reliability of a tool indicates its accuracy with respect to stability and repeatability in collecting data. In a paper-and-pencil test, for example, a test–retest method is commonly used to determine the test's reliability. That is, the test is given to a group similar to the group that will be studied, and, some time later, the test is readministered to the same group. Sufficient time must elapse between testing so that the memory of the test items is not fresh in the subjects' minds, but you must not leave so much time that there can be changes that might affect the subjects' responses the second time around. If the time conditions are right and if the test results remain the same or similar to those obtained the first time, the test is considered reliable. In other words, the reliability of an instrument is related to its ability to obtain the same data when repeated. Remember to expect some error or change, however, because the respondents are human beings and subject to the human frailty of unreliability.

Other methods of testing reliability include the alternate form test and the split-half or odd-even test of reliability. In the alternate form test, a two-part test is devised with each part containing similar questions and is administered to a group. To demonstrate reliability, the subjects must give similar answers in both parts of the test; in other words, one looks at the correlation of scores obtained from the two sets of questions. The split-half test for reliability involves only one set of questions, but two scores are obtained for comparison, one for the first half of the questions and one for the second half. The odd-even method also involves the use of two scores, but in this instance one is obtained from the answers to the odd-numbered questions and one from answers to the even-numbered questions. Another commonly used measure of internal consistency of an instrument is the Cronbach alpha coefficient. A reliability coefficient greater than 0.70 is usually evidence of adequate reliability.

Frequently, the tool to be used is tested in a pilot study, an important step in the development of a new tool. The purpose of the pilot study is to provide the researcher with information about the project that is planned. It should answer several questions: Is the project feasible (hence the name feasibility study)? Are the instruments reliable and valid for this population? Does the problem exist as it was proposed? Is the information obtainable in the way it was proposed? Many researchers find that starting with a pilot study it is an excellent way to "work out the kinks" in the plan. (See also exploratory study chapter 2.) We reiterate that, whenever possible, the novice researcher locate and use a tool, or a modification of one, that is already in existence and known to be valid and reliable.

Interrater reliability is the extent to which two or more independent judges are consistent in their observations, records, and scores from the same subject or subjects (see Hilton et al., 1990, for concise examples).

THE SAMPLE

In a quantitative study, a very important step in data collection is the selection of the sample, which is a representative selection of the group of the population to be studied. The sample must be consistent with the problem to be studied. In order for Budin (1998) to study psychosocial adjustment to breast cancer in unmarried women, the sample had to consist of women with breast cancer who were either single, separated, divorced, or widowed; she could not use a sample of married women or women with another health condition such as cardiac disease.

In addition, all characteristics to be studied must be represented in the sample. For example, in the classic study (Brooten et al., 1986) of early hospital discharge and home follow-up of infants with very low birth weight, the sample of mothers and infants were matched so that there were no statistically significant differences between the early discharge group and their controls in terms of the mother's age, educational level, marital status, race, or number of children; the family structure; the availability of a telephone in the home; the type of transportation available in an emergency; the family's reported annual income; the type of health insurance; or the number of children under 5 years of age. Between the experimental and the control groups of infants, there were no statistically significant differences in terms of infants' mean birth weight, gestational age, appropriateness of size for gestational age, number of days of ventilation, or number of days spent in the intensive care nursery.

The sample must also be representative of the total population of the group under study. Because it is frequently not possible to study the total population of, say, heroin addicts on all detoxification units, one settles for all the patients, or a sample of them, in one institution or in a group of institutions. If the sample is sufficiently large, it is assumed that the characteristics or phenomena observed will be representative of those that would be found in other groups. Replications of the same study in other institutions and in other parts of the country will establish representativeness.

Most current clinical research in nursing is limited to small, although representative, samples; therefore, generalizations to the total population can only be tentative. Brown (1990) and Beck (1990) both address this issue in their critiques, and Ford and Reutter (1990) point out the ethical dilemmas associated with small sample size in terms of "autonomy, non-maleficence, and beneficence" (pp. 187–190).

When the investigator plans to test a hypothesis by using certain statistical analyses of data or wishes to avoid bias in selection of the sample, what is known as a random sample is selected; that is, everyone in the group from which the sample is taken must have an equal chance or probability of being selected. In the study by Brooten et al. (1986) described previously, infants with birth weights of 1,500 g or less who were born at the Hospital of the University of Pennsylvania between October 1982 and December 1984 were randomly assigned to one of two groups. For other examples of random assignment of subjects, see Miller and Perry (1990) and Vessey et al. (1994); both studies were described in chapter 6.

A stratified random sample refers to a sample that has been randomized according to some added factor or factors, such as age, educational background, type of school, or perhaps religious affiliation. In the study testing the effects of a social support boosting intervention on stress, coping, and social support in caregivers of children with HIV/AIDS (Hansell et al., 1998), caregivers were stratified according to caregiver type (biological parents, foster parents, and extended family members) and then randomly assigned to experimental and control treatment groups.

A random sample can be obtained by putting slips containing the names of all possible subjects in a container, shaking the container well, and then withdrawing the required number of slips, one at a time. In order for this procedure to produce a truly random sample, each time a name is selected the slip is replaced in the container; if it comes up a second time, it is simply replaced again and another one drawn. In this way, every subject has an equal chance on each draw, and the question of selection bias is removed. Another method of making a random selection is to use a table of random numbers. (Tables of random numbers and explanations of their uses can be found in any standard text on statistics.) Computers are also useful for generating a list of random numbers.

A convenience sample is available and accessible to the researcher opportunistically, at the right place, at the right time, with the right demographics, and the right problem (e.g., AIDS, early postpartum discharge, breast cancer, post-CABG surgery) to be studied. Previously cited studies that also used convenience samples include Budin (1998); Hoskins et al. (1996); Redeker, Mason, Wykpisz, and Glica (1996); and Rentschler (1991).

SUMMARY

This chapter has presented information about a most important aspect of research: data collection. We have described a number of common methods of collecting data, methods of testing the validity and reliability of the instruments used in collecting and recording data, and the selection of an appropriate sample. Throughout this discussion, objectivity or freedom from bias was stressed. The next step in the research process, analyzing the collected data, will be presented in the following chapter.

REFERENCES

Aaronson, L., & Burman, M. (1994). Use of health records in research: Reliability and validity issues. *Research in Nursing and Health, 17,* 67–73.

Abdellah, F. G., & Levine, E. (1986). *Better patient care through nursing research* (3rd ed.). New York: Macmillan.

Beck, C. T. (1990). The research critique: General criteria for evaluating a research report. *Journal of Obstetric, Gynecologic and Neonatal Nursing, 19,* 18–22.

Beck, C. T. (1992). The lived experience of postpartum depression: A phenomenological study. *Nursing Research, 41,* 108–170.

Beck, C. T., Reynolds, M. A., & Rutowski, P. (1992). Maternity blues and postpartum depression. *Journal of Obstetric, Gynecologic and Neonatal Nursing, 21,* 287–293.

Brandt, P., & Weinert, C. (1987). The PRQ: A social support measure. *Nursing Research, 30,* 227–280.

Brennan, P., Moore, S., & Smyth, K. (1995). The effects of a special computer network on caregivers of persons with Alzheimer's disease. *Nursing Research, 44*(3), 166–172.

Brooten, D., Kumar, S., Brown, L. P., Butts, P., Finkler, S. A., Bakewell-Sachs, S., Gibbons, A., & Delivoria-Papadopoulos, M. (1986). A randomized clinical trial of early hospital discharge and home follow-up of very-low-birth-weight infants. *New England Journal of Medicine, 315,* 934–939.

Brown, S. A. (1990). Quality of reporting in diabetes patient education research: 1954–1986. *Research in Nursing and Health, 13,* 53–62.

Budin, W. (1998). Psychosocial adjustment to breast cancer in unmarried women. *Research in Nursing and Health, 21,* 155–166.

Burman, M. (1995). Health diaries in nursing research and practice. *Image: Journal of Nursing Scholarship, 27,* 147–152.

Burns, N., & Grove, S. (1997). *The practice of nursing research: Conduct, critique, & utilization* (3rd ed.). Philadelphia: W. B. Saunders.

Buros, O. (1998, February 18). *Buros Institute of Mental Measurements* [Online]. Available: http://www.unl.edu/buros/.

Butz, A., & Alexander, C. (1991). Use of health diaries with children. *Nursing Research, 40,* 59–61.

Camuñas, C., Alward, R. R., & Vecchione, E. (1990). Survey response rates to a professional association mail questionnaire. *Journal of the New York State Nurses Association, 21, 7–9.*

Carpenter, J. (1998). Informing participants about the benefits of descriptive research. *Nursing Research, 47,* 63–64.

Cohen, J., & Struening, E. (1963). Opinions about mental illness: Mental hospital occupational profiles and profile clusters. *Psychological Reports, 12,* 111–124.

Crisp, J., Pelletier, D., Duffield, C., Adams, A., & Nagy, S. (1997). The Delphi Method? *Nursing Research, 46,* 116–118.

Day, D., Hayes, K., Kennedy, A., & Diercksen, R. (1997). Pressure ulcer prevention: Review of the literature. *Journal of the New York State Nurses Association, 28,* 12–17.

Derogatis, L. (1983). *The Psychosocial Adjustment to Illness Scale.* Maryland: Clinical Psychometric Research.

Duffy, M. E. (1985). A research appraisal checklist for evaluating nursing research reports. *Nursing and Health Care, 6,* 539–547.

Engebretson, J. (1996). Comparison of nurses and alternative healers. *Image: Journal of Nursing Scholarship, 28,* 95–99.

Flaherty, J. A., Gaviria, F. M., & Pathak, D. S. (1983). The measurement of social support: The social support network inventory. *Comprehensive Psychiatry, 24,* 521–529.

Flaskerud, J. (1988). Is the Likert scale format culturally biased? *Nursing Research, 37,* 185–186.

Fitzpatrick, J. (1998). *Encyclopedia of nursing research.* New York: Springer Publishing Co.

Ford, J. S., & Reutter, L. I. (1990). Ethical dilemmas associated with small samples. *Journal of Advanced Nursing, 15,* 187–191.

Forte, P., Ritz, L., & Balestracci, D. (1997). Identifying nursing research priorities in a newly merged health care system. *Journal of Nursing Administration, 27,* 51–55.

Frank-Stromborg, M., & Olsen, S. (1997). *Instruments for clinical health-care research* (2nd ed.). Sudbury, MA: Jones and Bartlett.

Garrett, B. H. (1991). The relationship preferences, head nurse leader style, and job satisfaction of staff nurses. *Journal of the New York State Nurses Association, 22,* 11–14.

Gift, A. (1989). Visual analogue scales: Measurement of subjective phenomena. *Nursing Research, 38,* 286–288.

Goodridge, D. (1993). Pressure ulcer risk assessment tools: What's new for gerontological nurses. *Journal of Geronlogical Nursing, 19,* 23–27.

Gordon, S., & Stokes, S. (1989). Improving response rate to mailed questionnaires. *Nursing Research, 38,* 375–376.

Hansell, P., Hughes, C., Caliandro, G., Russo, P., Budin, W., Hartman, B., & Hernandez, O. (1998). The effects of a social support boosting intervention on stress, coping, and social support in caregivers of children with HIV/AIDS. *Nursing Research, 47,* 79–86.

HaPI. (1998). *Health and Psychosocial Instruments.* Behavioral Measurement Database Service, PO Box 1100287, Pittsburgh, PA.

Heacock, P., Souder, E., & Chastain, J. (1996). Subjects, data, and videotapes. *Nursing Research, 45,* 336–338.

Heitkemper, M., Jarrett, M., Bond, E., & Turner, P. (1991). GI symptoms, function, and psychophysiological arousal in dysmenorrheic women. *Nursing Research, 40,* 20–26.

Hilton, G., Sisson, R., & Freeman, E. (1990). The neurobehavioral rating scale: An interrator reliability study in the HIV seropositive population. *Journal of Neuroscience Nursing, 22,* 36–42.

Hoskins, C., Baker, S., Budin, W., Ekstrom, D., Maislin, G., Sherman, D., Steelman-Bohlander, J., Bookbinder, M., & Knauer, C. (1996). Adjustment among husbands of women with breast cancer. *Journal of Psychosocial Oncology, 14,* 41–69.

Hutchinson, S., & Wilson, H. S. (1992). Validity threats in scheduled semistructured research interviews. *Nursing Research, 41,* 117–119.

Hutchinson, S., Wilson, M., & Wilson, H. (1994). Benefits of participating in research interviews. *Image: Journal of Nursing Scholarship, 26,* 161–164.

Iglesias, G. (1998). Role evolution of the mental health clinical nurse specialist in home care. *Clinical Nurse Specialist, 12,* 38–44.

Jones, E. G., & Kay, M. (1992). Instrumentation in cross-cultural research. *Nursing Research, 41,* 186–188.

Keane, M. (1991). Beliefs about mental illness in a culturally diverse nursing student population: Implications for education and practice. *Journal of the New York State Nurses Association, 22,* 15–18.

Kemp, V. H. (1990). Selecting instruments in research. *NAACOG Newsletter, 17,* 9, 14.

Killion, C. (1995). Special health needs of homeless pregnant women. *Advances in Nursing Science, 18(2),* 44–56.

Link, B., McNamara, R., Penney, D., & Ungemack, J. (1978). *The measurement of attitudes towards the mentally ill in group homes.* Unpublished manuscript.

Lorig. K., Gonzalez, V., Ritter, P., & DeBrey, V. (1997). Comparison of three methods of data collection in an urban Spanish-speaking population. *Nursing Research, 46,* 230–234.

Lothian, J. (1995). It takes two to breastfeed: The baby's role in successful breastfeeding. *Journal of Nurse-Midwifery, 40,* 328–334.

Mariano, C. (1990). Qualitative research. *Nursing and Health Care, 11,* 354–359.

McCorkle, R., & Young, K. (1978). Development of a symptom distress scale. *Cancer Nursing, 1,* 373–378.

Micelli, D., Waxman, H., Cavalieri, T., & Lage, S. (1994). Prodromal falls among older nursing home residents. *Applied Nursing Research, 7,* 18–27.

Miller, K. M., & Perry, P. A. (1990). Relaxation technique and postoperative pain in patients undergoing cardiac surgery. *Heart and Lung: Journal of Critical Care, 19,* 136–146.

Minnick, A., Roberts, M., Young, W., Kleinpell, R., & Micek, W. (1995). An analysis of posthospitilization telephone survey data. *Nursing Research, 44,* 371–375.

Misener, T., Alexander, J., Blaha, A., Clark, P., Cover, C., Felton, G., Fuller, S., Herman, J., Rodes, M., & Sharp, H. (1997). National Delphi study to determine competencies for nursing leadership in public health. *Image: Journal of Nursing Scholarship, 29*(1), 47–51.

Murphy, G. (1994). *Psychosocial adjustment to illness: An examination of measures.* Unpublished doctoral dissertation, New York University, NY.

Nappier, P., Stanfield, J., Simon, J. M., Bennett, S., & Gowan, C. F. (1990). Identifying clinical research priorities. *Nursing Connections, 3,* 45–50.

Oleske, D., Heinze, S., & Otte, D. (1990). The diary as a means of understanding the quality of persons with cancer receiving home nursing care. *Cancer Nursing, 13,* 158–166.

Olshansky, E. (1987). Infertility and career identities. *Health Care for Women International, 8,* 185–196.

Olshansky, E. (1990). Psychosocial implications of pregnancy after infertility. *Journal of Obstetric, Gynecologic and Neonatal Nursing, 1,* 342–347.

Olshansky, E. (1996). Theoretical issues in building a grounded theory: Application of an example of a program of research on infertility. *Qualitative Health Research, 6*(3), 394–405.

Pill, J. (1970). *The Delphi Method: Substance, context, a critique and an annotated bibliography* (Technical Memorandum No. 183). Cleveland, OH: Operations Research Department, School of Management, Case Western Reserve University.

Polit, D. F., & Hungler, B. P. (1995). *Nursing research: Principles and methods* (5th ed.). Philadelphia: Lippincott.

Pugh, L., & DeKeyser, F. (1995). Use of physiologic variables in nursing research. *Image, 27,* 273–276.

Redeker, N., Mason, D., Wykpisz, E., & Glica, B. (1996). Sleep patterns in women after coronary artery bypass surgery. *Applied Nursing Research, 9,* 115–122.

Rentschler, D. (1991). Correlates of successful breastfeeding. *Nursing Research, 23,* 151–154.

Roberts, B., Srour, M., & Winkelman, C. (1996). Videotaping: An important research strategy. *Nursing Research, 45,* 334–338.

Schmidt, K., Montgomery, L., Bruene, D., & Kenney, M. (1997). Determining research priorities in pediatric nursing: A Delphi study. *Journal of Pediatric Nursing, 12,* 201–207.

Schroeder, C. (1996). Women's experience of bed rest in high-risk pregnancy. *Image, 28,* 253–258.

Seideman, R. (1990). Effects of premenstrual syndrome education program on premenstrual symptomatology. *Health Care for Women International, 11,* 491–505.

Sherman, D. (1996). Nurses' willingness to care for AIDS patients and spirituality, social support, and death anxiety. *Image, 28,* 205–213.

Skrutkowska, M., & Weijer, C. (1997). Do patients with breast cancer participating in clinical trials receive better care? *Oncology Nursing Forum, 24,* 1411–1416.

Snyder, M. (1989). Valid, reliable, and usable measurement. *Nursing Scan in Research: Application for Clinical Practice, 2,* 1–3.

Strickland, O., Hinshaw, A. S., & DiLorio, C. (Eds.). (1998). *Journal of Nursing Measurement.* New York: Springer Publishing Co.

Taussig, J. E., & Freeman, E. W. (1988). The next best thing to being there: Conducting the clinical research interview by telephone. *American Journal of Orthopsychiatry, 58,* 418–426.

Templer, D. (1970). The construction and validation of a death anxiety scale. *Journal of General Psychology, 82,* 165–177.

Toseland, R., & Rossiter, C. (1989). Group interventions to support family caregivers: A review and analysis. *Gerontologist, 29,* 438–477.

Van Servellen, G., Lewis, C., & Leake, B. (1990). The stresses of hospitalization among AIDS patients on integrated special care units. *International Journal of Nursing Studies, 27,* 235–247.

Vessey, J., Carlson, K., & McGill, J. (1994). Use of distraction with children during an acute pain experience. *Nursing Research, 43,* 369–372.

Volicer, B., & Bohannon, M. (1975). A hospital stress rating. *Nursing Research, 24,* 352–364.

von Essen, L., & Sjoden, P. (1993). Perceived importance of caring behaviors to Swedish psychiatric inpatients and staff, with comparisons to somatically-ill samples. *Research in Nursing and Health, 16,* 293–303.

Von Post, I. (1996). Exploring ethical dilemmas in perioperative nursing practice through critical incidents. *Nursing Ethics: An International Journal, 3,* 236–249.

Wagnild, G., & Young, H. (1990). Resilience among older women. *Image: Journal of Nursing Scholarship, 22,* 252–255.

Waltz, C., Strickland, O., & Lenz, E. (1991). *Measurement in nursing research.* Philadelphia: F. A. Davis.

Waltz, C., & Strickland, O. (Eds.). (1988a). *Measuring client outcomes* (Vol. 1). New York: Springer Publishing Co.

Waltz, C., & Strickland, O. (Eds.). (1988b). *Measuring nursing performance practice, education, and research* (Vol. 2). New York: Springer Publishing Co.

Waltz, C., & Strickland, O. (Eds.). (1990). *Measuring clinical skills and professional development in education and practice* (Vol. 3). New York: Springer Publishing Co.

Waltz, C., & Strickland, O. (Eds.). (1991). *Measuring client self-care and coping skills* (Vol. 4). New York: Springer Publishing Co.

Williams, P., & Webb, C. (1994). The Delphi technique: A methodological discussion. *Journal of Advanced Nursing, 19,* 180–186.

Wingate, A., & Lackey, N. (1989). A description of the needs of noninstitutionalized cancer patients and their primary caregivers. *Cancer Nursing, 12,* 216–225.

Wong, D., & Baker, C. (1988). Pain in children's comparison of assessment scales. *Pediatric Nursing, 14,* 9–17.

Woods, N. F., Taylor, D., Mitchell, E. S., & Lentz, M. J. (1992). Perimenstrual symptoms and health-seeking behavior. *Western Journal of Nursing Research, 14,* 418–443.

Woods, N. F., Olshansky, E., & Draye, M. (1991). Infertility: Women's experiences. *Health Care for Women International, 12,* 179–190.

8

Analysis of the Data

For an investigator to make a meaningful analysis of the data collected in a study, the methods used to collect it must be appropriate to the study of the problem being investigated. The research question you ask and the type of data you collect determine the method of data analysis for your study. For example, Rentschler (1991) studied the factors related to success in breast-feeding. Pregnant women's achievement motivation, as measured by a prenatal questionnaire, or prenatal information about breast-feeding in a questionnaire, and a personal data inventory that were followed by a breast-feeding questionnaire 6 weeks postpartum, were the data-collection tools. They became the data to determine the relationship Rentschler was questioning.

The method of analyzing data that is selected for a study involves knowing in advance how the data are to be summarized and interpreted. There are three very simple reasons why the investigator must think through what the method of analysis will be at the time decisions are made about the method of collecting data: The investigator must determine (1) what data to collect, (2) how to collect them, and (3) whether one can collect them at all. For example, in the Rentschler (1991) study, all the variables had to be determined in advance so that data on them would be available for the kind of analysis the investigator had planned. The beginning investigator who does not study the situation carefully enough during the planning stage can find that when coming to the stage of analysis, some of the necessary information has not been collected. There is no question about it: The more time spent in planning all phases of the study, the better the chances of ending up with a well-designed study.

At the outset, let us emphasize that the object of this chapter is not to teach you statistics. Duffy (1988) says, "Statistics is an area of mathematics that seeks to make order out of a large array of diverse facts or data" (p. 73), making the point that many are concerned with statistics because they are seen as an end in themselves, rather than as the means to an end, which they are. So look at this as a "reader-friendly" chapter. Statistics are not your enemy. This chapter is meant as an introduction to methods of grouping and analyzing data and to some of the concepts basic to statistical approaches.

CLASSIFYING AND ORGANIZING THE DATA

Once data are collected, they must be organized and displayed in a fashion that will help the researcher to understand them. The data for a research study may be either qualitative or quantitative. The Schroeder (1996) study, mentioned in chapters 6 and 7, used qualitative methods, and the findings were presented as examples of passages from the interviews that captured the essence of the themes identified. No numerical data were presented. Another example of the presentation of qualitative data is shown in Table 8.1. In this table, Beck (1992, p. 168) provides selected examples of significant statements and corresponding formulated meanings from her phenomenological study of the lived experience of postpartum depression.

Whereas the data in a qualitative study are usually presented in the form of words, the data in a quantitative study are presented in terms of numbers representing facts. The remainder of this chapter will focus on the analysis of quantitative data. One can begin by grouping like facts together. If the data include scores of a group on a test, they can be tallied somewhat as follows:

Scores	Tally	Totals
100		
99	/	1
98		
97	//	2
96		
95	/////	5
etc.		

In other words, having like scores grouped together gives one a clearer, more concise picture of the data. The data collected in the study by Hansell et al. (1998) on caregivers of children with HIV/AIDS were mainly quantitative in nature. Some of the data, which were collected on sample characteristics according to caregiver HIV status, were grouped to facilitate analysis of their meaning and presented in tabular form. Table 8.2 provides a breakdown of ethnic background, marital status, educational level, and social status according to the Hollingshead Index.

TABLE 8.1 Presentation of Qualitative Data. Selected Examples of Significant Statements of Postpartum Depression and Corresponding Formulated Meanings

Significant statements	Formulated meanings
1. I was very suicidal because there was no way anyone could endure the kind of pain I was going through.	1. Suicidal thoughts prevailed as her quality of life became intolerable.
2. You want to be okay and you try, but the fogginess and fatigue would set in.	2. Attempts to overcome the depression were hindered by the fogginess and fatigue.
3. I was like a baby because I had to be taken care of and couldn't be left alone.	3. She perceived she had regressed to an infancy state where she was incapable of taking care of herself.
4. I would think, not that I would hurt my baby, but what if I didn't intervene to help him or to give him something.	4. She was horrified by her thoughts of not intervening to help her baby if he needed her.
5. I would lie awake at night having a lot of obsessive thinking.	5. She was haunted by obsessive thoughts while trying to fall asleep.

Note. From "The lived experience of postpartum depression: A phenomenological study," by C. T. Beck, 1992, *Nursing Research, 41,* p. 168.

As can be seen in Table 8.2, both actual numbers and percentages are reported for the variables for the total sample. This is a good procedure because it allows the reader to see at a glance what the percentages really mean. It is of the utmost importance that this procedure be adhered to when small numbers are involved. With small numbers the use of percentages alone may be misleading.

Table 8.3 shows a method of ranking data. In this study by Pettengill, Gillies, and Clark (1994, p. 146), 182 nurses working in education and 222 nurses working in nursing service were asked to rank order the factors that discouraged them from using nursing research findings in practice. Lack of time was most discouraging to educators and service nurses. The second strongest discourager for educators was lack of support from nursing administration, whereas for service nurses it was lack of nursing staff support. Lack of support from other health disciplines was also a discourager for both service and educator nurses. The least important discourager for both service and educator nurses was prior negative experience with research activities in practice or education.

Most of the simple evaluative studies in which you may be involved will be descriptive and will require grouping of data by frequencies and percentages or rankings, whether by scores, tallies of questionnaire

TABLE 8.2 Data Grouped by Frequencies and Percentages. Sample Characteristics According to Caregiver HIV Status

	Seronegative ($n = 31$)	Seropositive ($n = 39$)	Total sample ($n = 70$)	
Variable	*n*	*n*	*n*	%
Ethnic background				
African American	26	25	51	73
White	5	4	9	13
Hispanic	7	2	9	13
Marital status				
Single	18	9	27	39
Separated/divorced	7	11	18	26
Widowed	2	2	4	5
Partnered	8	1	9	13
Married	4	8	12	17
Educational level				
< Seventh grade	2	0	2	3
Junior HS	6	2	8	11
Partial HS	14	5	19	27
HS graduate	8	6	14	20
Partial college	8	12	20	29
College graduate	1	6	7	10
Hollingshead Index				
Social Status 1	26	5	31	44
Social Status 2	6	12	18	26
Social Status 3	7	8	15	22
Social Status 4	0	2	2	3
Social Status 5	0	3	3	4
Missing data			1	1

Note. From "The effects of a social support boosting intervention on stress, coping, and social support in caregivers of children with HIV/AIDS," by Hansell et al., 1998, *Nursing Research, 47*(2), p. 81.

answers, or enumerations of observations made. In more complex descriptive studies and in experimental research, more sophisticated groupings may be made. For example, averages or mean scores rather than the actual scores may be grouped for analysis, as was done in the study on the effects of a social support boosting intervention on stress, coping, and social support in caregivers of children with HIV/AIDS (Hansell et al., 1998) (see Table 8.4 and Figure 8.1).

In Table 8.4 the mean scores for the variables stress, coping, and social support are listed for the total sample, the experimental group, and the control group at two data collection points. Along with the

TABLE 8.3 Rank Ordering of Factors that Discourage Research Utilization. What Discourages You From Using Nursing Research Findings in Your Practice? Rankings (most to least important)

Sample	1st	2nd	3rd	4th	5th	6th	7th	8th
Education ($n = 182$)	Time	Lack nursing admin. support and others	Lack of interest nursing staff	Lack support others	Lack support others	Negative experience in education	Negative experience in practice	Negative experience in education
Service ($n = 222$)	Time	Lack of interest nursing staff	Lack support others	Lack support others	Lack support others	Negative experience in practice	Lack nursing admin. support	Negative experience in practice

Note. From "Factors encouraging and discouraging use of nursing research findings," by M. Pettengill et al., 1994, *Image: Journal of Nursing Scholarship*, *26*(2), p. 146.

TABLE 8.4 Data Grouped by Mean Scores in a Table. Descriptive Statistics for Stress, Coping, and Social Support at Baseline (DC1) and 6 Months (DC2) for Total Sample and Experimental and Control Groups

	DC1			DC2		
	X	*SD*	Range	X	*SD*	Range
Total sample ($n = 70$)						
Stress	529.0	(73.4)	263–665	530.0	(54.6)	423–665
Coping	106.0	(16.6)	70–142	106.0	(14.6)	68–138
Social support	4.1	(0.6)	2.0–5.0	3.9	(0.66)	1.7–5.0
Experimental group ($n = 34$)						
Stress	513.0	(68.7)	364–661	520.0	(50.9)	423–612
Coping	104.0	(16.4)	70–138	105.0	(12.9)	70–129
Social support	4.23	(0.57)	1.7–4.9	4.07	(0.7)	1.7–4.9
Control group ($n = 36$)						
Stress	544.0	(75.6)	263–665	540.0	(56.9)	431–665
Coping	108.0	(16.78)	74–142	106.0	(16.2)	68–138
Social support	4.04	(0.62)	2.7–5.0	3.91	(0.62)	2.7–5.0

Note. Stress was measured by the total score of the Derogatis Stress Profile. Coping was measured by the total score of the F-COPES, and Social Support was measured by the interpersonal support scale of the Tilden Interpersonal Relationship Inventory. From "The effects of a social support boosting intervention on stress, coping, and social support in caregivers of children with HIV/AIDS," by P. Hansell et al., 1998, *Nursing Research, 47*(2), p. 83.

mean scores are the standard deviation and the range of scores for each variable (Hansell et al., 1998, p. 83).

Figure 8.1 provides an example of how mean scores can be shown in a graph. This example, also from the study on caregivers of children with HIV/AIDS, shows changes in mean social support levels over time. The key provided in the table at the bottom of the graph identifies four groups of caregivers: seropositive caregivers in the experimental group, seronegative caregivers in the experimental group, seropositive caregivers in the control group, and seronegative caregivers in the control group. Looking at the graph one can see that the only group of caregivers that showed an increase in levels of social support over time was the seronegative caregivers in the experimental group. These researchers (Hansell et al., 1998, p. 85) concluded that seronegative caregivers derived substantial benefit from the social support boosting intervention.

Figure 8.2 provides another example of how mean scores can be displayed on graph. In this study, Cusson, Madonia, and Taekman (1997, p. 205), tested the effect of environment on temperature by comparing

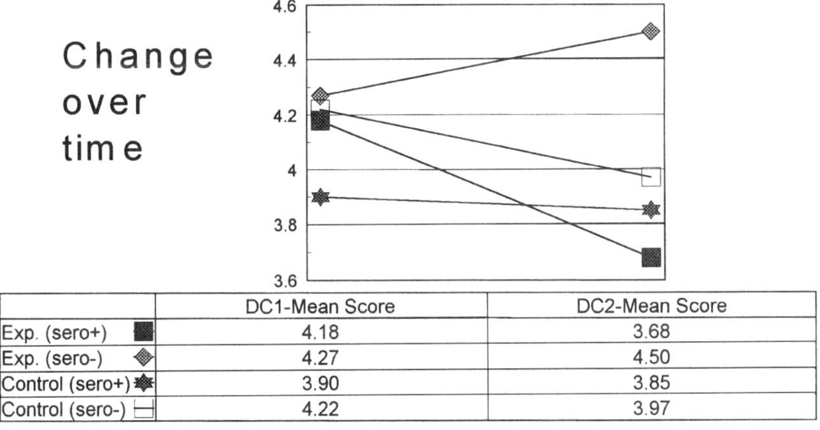

	DC1-Mean Score	DC2-Mean Score
Exp. (sero+)	4.18	3.68
Exp. (sero-)	4.27	4.50
Control (sero+)	3.90	3.85
Control (sero-)	4.22	3.97

$F(1,66) = 10.39, p = .002$

FIGURE 8.1 Graph of mean scores showing change over time. Changes in mean social support levels over time (DC1 = baseline, DC2 = 6 months).

Note. From "The effects of a social support boosting intervention on stress, coping, and social support in caregivers of children with HIV/AIDS," by P. Hansell et al., 1998, *Nursing Research, 47*(2), p. 85.

tympanic, rectal, inguinal, and axillary temperatures for 63 term infants in three environments: incubator, bassinet, and radiant warmer. Examining the graph one can see that the environment seems to influence temperature readings at the different sites. Temperatures assessed in the superheated environments of the radiant warmer and the incubator were consistently higher than temperatures in the bassinet were.

Data that have been collected must be organized in some fashion so that they can be analyzed and so that the investigator can arrive at a statement of results. As we noted previously, data can be organized in a variety of ways for inspection and analysis in order to give the researcher as much information as possible. Hansell et al. (1998) organized their data according to such variables as stress, coping, and social support, HIV status of the caregiver, and data collection time; Pettengill et al. (1994) organized their data by factors that discourage research use, and the ranks assigned by nurses in both education and service; and Cusson et al. (1997) organized their data according to temperature site and environment.

The reason for organizing data for analysis is to make manifest possible relationships, proportions, trends, or tendencies; that is, to reveal the nature of the information that has been gathered. For example, there may be sex differences or differences related to age. Hansell et al.

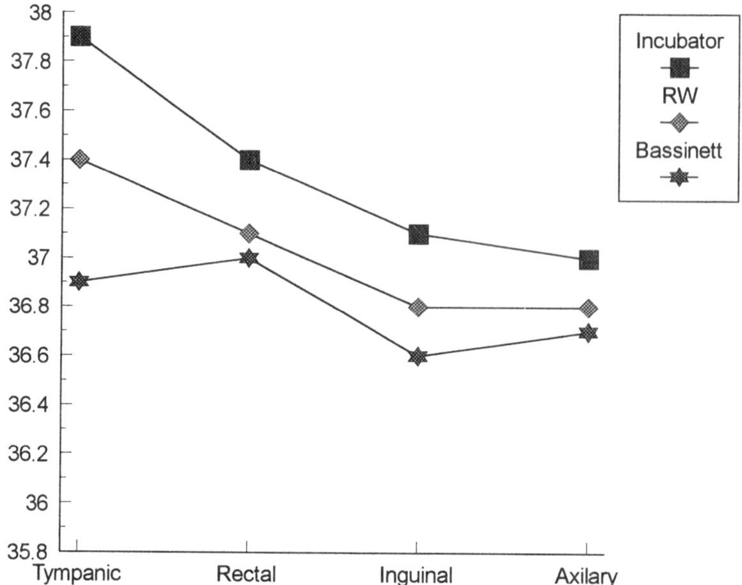

FIGURE 8.2 Graph of mean scores for temperature. Mean temperature by site and environment.

Note. From "The effect of environment on body site temperature in full-term neonates," by R. Cusson et al., 1997, *Nursing Research, 46*(4), p. 205.

found that the seronegative caregivers were significantly older ($M = 42$ years) than the seropositive caregivers were ($M = 32$ years) ($t = -5.2$, $p < 0.001$). The seronegative caregivers were also of a higher educational level and a higher social status. No differences were noted in racial background or marital status between the seropositive and seronegative caregivers, however.

When data are presented in tabular form it is important that they be adequately and properly labeled. Each table should have a title that describes its contents and should be set up with both vertical and horizontal columns. Each row and column should have a heading that describes the information in the respective row or column. In the tables shown in this chapter, the titles are descriptive of the table contents, and each row and column is carefully identified. (For a more detailed discussion of how to set up tables, see Publication Manual of the American Psychological Association [1994].)

Graphs and bar charts or pictorial charts may be used to present data. This kind of graphic and dramatic picture of relationships will give the information more quickly than a table of frequencies (see Figures 8.3 and 8.4).

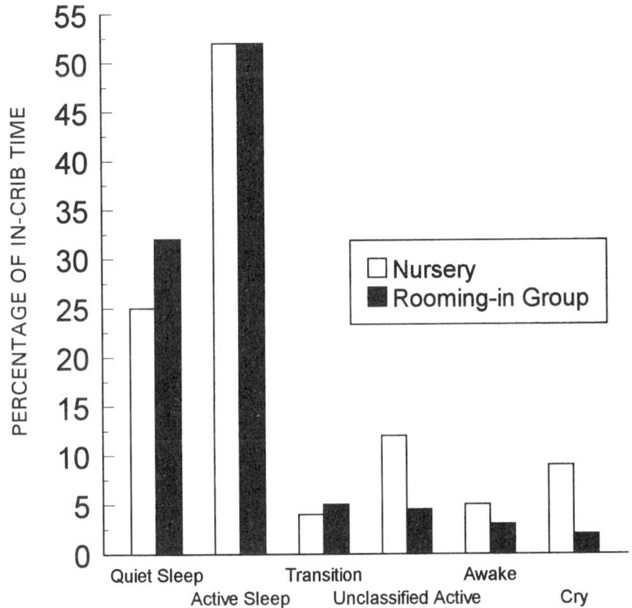

FIGURE 8.3 An example bar chart. Group differences in state: Nursery vs. rooming-in.

Note. From "Comparison of neonatal nighttime sleep-wake patterns in nursery versus rooming-in environments," by M. R. Keefe, 1987, *Nursing Research, 36,* p. 143.

Figure 8.3 is a simple bar chart showing group differences in sleep-wake states between babies in a nursery and those in a rooming-in environment (Keefe, 1987, p. 143). A quick glance at this chart will allow the reader to see that babies in the nursery group were awake more and seemed to cry more than did babies who were rooming in with their mothers.

Figure 8.4 is a creative pictorial histogram showing distribution by racial ethnic group of the RN population as compared with the U.S. population (Trossman, 1998). By glancing at these figures one can see that the RN population does not mirror the U.S. population. Nearly 90% of the total RN population is White, compared with roughly 72% of the total U.S. population. A pictorial histogram is worth a thousand words.

STATISTICAL ANALYSIS OF DATA

In addition to using simple enumeration, grouping, and inspection in analyzing collected information, statistical analysis may be used. This

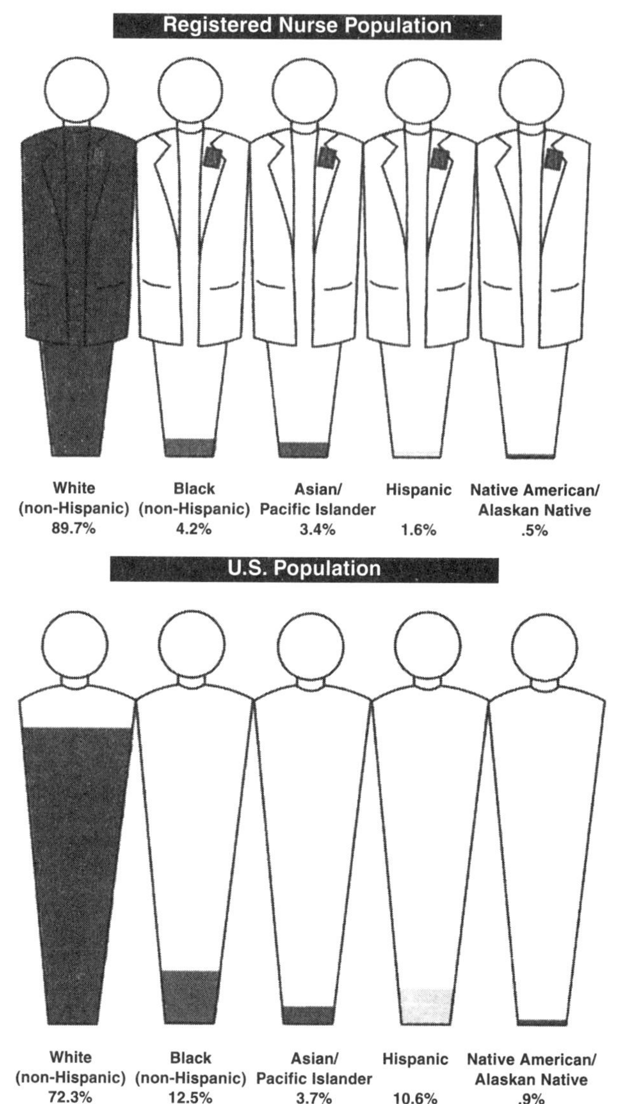

FIGURE 8.4 Pictorial histogram. Distribution by racial/ethnic group—March 1996.

Note. From "Nursing profession must mirror society's diversity," by S. Trossman, 1998, *The American Nurse, 30*(1), p. 25.

includes such measures of central tendency as means, medians, modes, and standard deviation *(SD)*, as well as more sophisticated measures, to estimate the chances that the findings can be generalized to the larger population.

If you are conducting a quantitative study that requires the use of statistics and you have not had special preparation in this area, you should consult a statistician or experienced researcher about this phase of your study. You should do this before you start to collect the data to ensure the data you collect are appropriate for the statistics you plan to use. You should also seek a statistician's help in organizing the data, computing the statistics, analyzing the results of the computation, and deciding on the correct method of reporting the findings. Many universities and other institutions have consultants available to assist with data management and statistical analysis. If you are not conducting a study, it is still important that you have a basic understanding of statistical procedures so you can interpret the findings of a study and be an informed consumer of nursing research.

Descriptive Statistics

A variety of statistical procedures are commonly used in quantitative descriptive studies, correlational studies, and experimental research in which the findings on groups are compared or relationships are described. Statistics that describe data include some methods we have already mentioned: frequency distribution or grouping of the raw data. Data can be measured on a nominal, ordinal, interval, or ratio scale.

Nominal data consist of categories or names of discrete factors, such as gender, race, or nursing specialty. Code numbers assigned to levels of these factors have no numerical value. For example, a researcher who wished to categorize the variable gender might assign the following codes: 1 = male, 2 = female. One cannot interpret these numbers to say that females have more "gender" than males. With nominal data, code numbers are used only for grouping purposes. No statistical procedures other than calculating percentages can be performed on nominal data. In other words, it would be meaningless to calculate a mean or average gender of a sample.

Ordinal data are categories of data placed in relative order on the basis of some specific criterion, for example, ranking of the importance of some factor such as various teaching strategies from least important to most important. Level of education might also be measured on an ordinal scale where 1 = elementary school, 2 = middle school, 3 = high school, 4 = college, and 5 = graduate school. As you can see in this example the code numbers assigned have an order that tells the relative ranking. For example, someone with a college education (4) has a higher level of education than someone with a middle school education (2). One cannot say, however, that someone with a college education has twice the level of education as someone with a middle school education. The intervals between the categories are not assumed to be equal. This limits the type of statistical procedures that can be performed with ordinal data.

Interval data are measured on a scale on which the values can be ranked and the numerical distance or interval between values are equal. For example, temperature readings, such as 98.6, 98.7, 98.8, and so on, are reported at the intervals noted. In this example, the difference between a temperature of 98.6 and 99.6 is the same as the difference between a temperature of 99.6 and 100.6.

Ratio level data are the highest level of measurement. Ratio scales are similar to interval scales in that the values can be ranked and the intervals between values are equal. In a ratio scale, however, there is a fixed zero, indicating the absence of the property being measured.

When a researcher uses data measured on an interval or ratio scale, the number of statistical procedures that can be used increases considerably. A comparison of ratio, interval, ordinal, and nominal data is provided in Munro (1997) and Polit-O'Hara (1996).

To describe quantitative data we may wish to show a range, for example, the range of scores on a test before and after some treatment or course. We may also want to show measures of central tendency, such as the mean, median, and mode. The mean (an average) is obtained by adding all the scores and dividing the sum by the total number of scores. The median is the exact middle score and is obtained by separating the scores into upper and lower halves. The mode is the score that occurs most frequently.

Measures of variability also provide a good picture of the data. The range is the distance between the top and bottom scores; it is the simplest measure of variability. The *SD* is a frequently used statistic that shows how scores will vary about the mean. Methods of computing the SD can be found in any basic text on statistics. It is derived by taking the square root of the variance, which is the average of the sum of squares of all scores in the distribution. Figure 8.5 shows the *SD* for data that follow the normal curve. The normal curve is a distribution in which mean, median, and mode coincide on the same point. When distribution is normal, 68.2% of the scores will fall between –1 and +1 *SD* from the mean, 95.4% will fall between –2 and +2 *SD*, and 99.8% of the scores will fall between –3 and +3 *SD* from the mean.

Knowing measures of central tendency and measures of variability may be important to know, particularly if the distribution of scores is

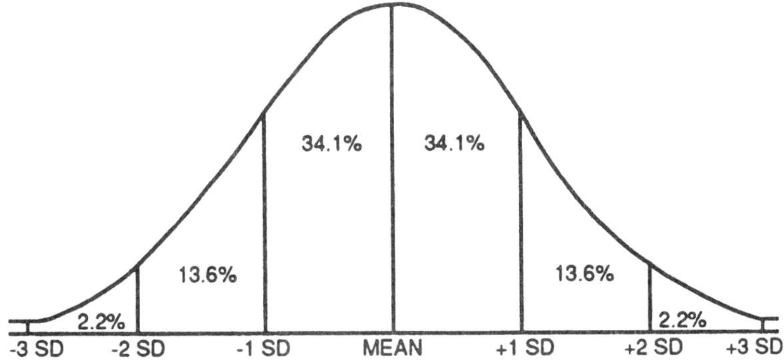

FIGURE 8.5 The normal curve and standard deviations.

skewed in some way. When a distribution is positively skewed, it means that the bulk of the scores fall in the lower range, below the mean, and the tail of the distribution extends toward the higher values. When a distribution is negatively skewed it means that the bulk of the scores are above the mean and the tail of the distribution extends toward the lower scores (Figure 8.6). Outliers, or extreme values, may skew a distribution of scores.

Another way of showing relationships is through the use of correlation procedures. Correlations show either a positive or a negative relationship. A –1 relationship indicates a perfect negative or inverse relationship between two groups or variables studied; a +1 relationship indicates that they show a perfect positive relationship. That is, in the first case (–1), when the value of one variable goes up the value of the other variable goes down; in the second case (+1), when the value of one variable goes up the value of the other goes up also. A 0 correlation indicates no relationship at all. Of course, there are gradations between –1, 0, and +1. These are always expressed as parts of 1; for example, 0.80, 0.70, 0.10, and so on.

Bivariate correlations show a relationship between two variables. This relationship may be positive and fairly high, thus increasing the chance that when one occurs the other is likely to be present. Multiple correlations show relationship among more than two variables. It is important to point out that relationships measured with correlational statistics can never be interpreted as a causal, meaning that a change in one causes a change in the other. Correlational statistics are particularly useful in answering such questions as

- What is the relationship between *x* and y?
- To what extent can variables *A, B,* and *C* explain variable *D*?
- To what extent can variables *A, B,* and *C* explain/relate to variables *D, E,* and *F*?

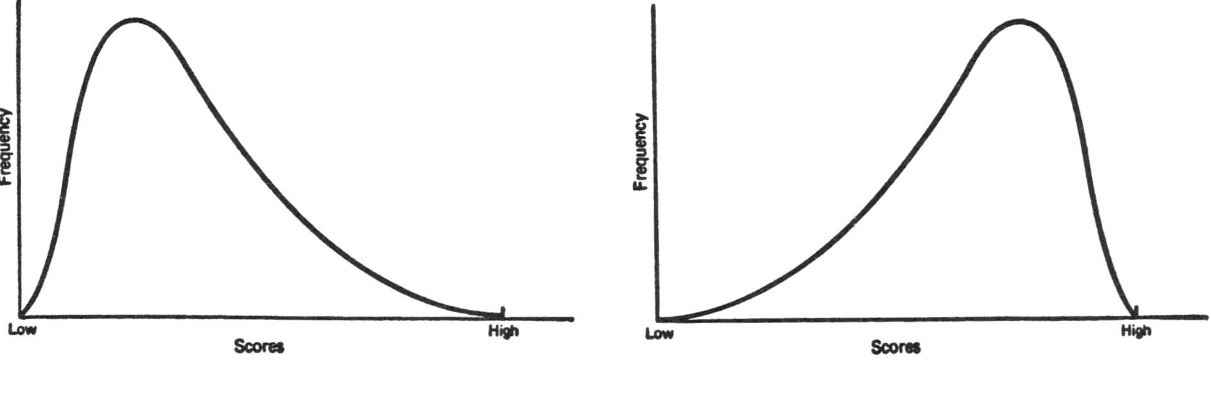

Positive skew **Negative skew**

FIGURE 8.6 Skewed distributions.

Statistical Inference

In addition to the use of descriptive statistics, which summarize and describe numerical data, the investigator may use inferential statistics to make inferences whether an observed relationship or an observed difference is statistically significant. For example, we might consider the hypothetical study discussed in chapter 3, the comparison of effectiveness of two methods of teaching diabetic patients self-care: group instruction versus individual computerized instruction. If you found that the group having computerized instruction scored higher on the measurements used, you would want to know whether the difference in the data obtained was significantly different or merely due to chance. In order to determine whether a difference observed is a significant one, a statistical test of significance is used. These tests have been developed to help us estimate the probability of the difference being due to chance. If we found that patients with computerized instruction performed better than those receiving group instruction, we would have to consider that this occurred by chance; that is, the group in our sample may have done better this time, but if the experiment were to be repeated a number of times, we might find that, on the average, there was no difference between the two methods of teaching.

The probability of chance has often been likened to the toss of a coin. Because a coin has two sides, there is a 50-50 chance on each toss that heads will show up. One seldom observes that heads will come up at every other toss, however. It is more likely that some other combination will occur when one tosses the coin several times. The probability of the number of times heads will appear in relation to the number of throws, however, can be calculated. If, for some reason, heads appear more often or less often than the calculated probability of chance, there is something else explaining the significant difference. We have no trick coins in research. It is important to understand the function of probability and chance in looking for facts or testing theories in nursing, as well as in all scientific studies. The level of difference we will accept in deciding what is significant is based on the concepts of probability and chance.

The level of significance refers to the probability that the difference between sets of data is due to chance. The investigator sets the probability level that will be accepted at the time the research is designed. For example, a researcher may decide to accept a probability (p) of 0.01. This $p = 0.01$ or $p < 0.01$ (which sets the probability at 1% or less than 1%) means that results would occur by chance less than 1% of the time, or only 1 time out of every 100. Acceptable levels of significance are usually 0.01 or 0.05. If the significant difference turns out to be greater than 0.05, say 0.10 or 0.20, there would be too great a probability that the difference observed was due to chance, and the investigator would report that there was no significant difference. These tests of significance are particularly useful in analyzing the data in relation to the hypothesis made at the beginning of the study. The null hypothesis, you will remember, states that no difference or no relationship will be found. If the null hypothesis is rejected, the researcher supports or accepts the alternative, that there is a significant difference or significant relationship. If the null hypothesis is accepted, then no significant difference or relationship was found.

There are a number of inferential statistics used to test hypotheses. The choice will depend on the type of data that are collected, the purpose of the study, the design, and the hypotheses being tested or the research questions being answered. The chi-square is a frequently used statistical test when the data collected are nominal or consist of frequencies in discrete categories. Chi-square compares the actual number, or observed frequency, in each group with the expected number or frequency. Chi-square can be used to analyze differences among groups. An example of the use of chi-square can be seen in Horns, Ratcliffe, Leggett, and Swanson (1996, p. 51). The purpose of this study was to compare pregnancy outcomes between sedentary and active primiparous women. Prior to comparing pregnancy outcomes, the characteristics of the women in the sedentary and active groups were compared using chi-square statistics. Table 8.5 illustrates summaries for the chi-square analysis. The table shows that participants were similar in terms of ethnicity, marital status, and age. The active group had significantly more education, 38% with postbachelor's education, compared with 9% in the sedentary group. Cesarean birth rates were high in both groups, with rates of 32% and 25% in the sedentary and active groups, respectively. Data for chi-square analyses are often presented in contingency tables. A contingency table visibly identifies an association of data within selected combinations of categories.

The *t*-test is a statistical procedure that is used to test the differences between the means of two groups. It is based on the *t*-distribution, which is different from the normal curve shown in Figure 8.4. In the *t*-distribution, the smaller the sample, the flatter the curve, with proportionally more cases distributed at the ends of the curve. An example of the use of the *t*-test to measure results can be seen in Table 8.6 (Horns, 1996, p. 53). The table presents the tests of significance for differences between the sedentary group and the active group on the selected pregnancy outcome variables. Examining Table 8.6, one can see that no significant differences were found between the two groups on mean weight gain during pregnancy, infant birth weight, gestational age, or number of discomforts. For participants delivering vaginally, no significant differences

TABLE 8.5 Example of Chi-Square Results. Characteristics of the Women in the Sedentary and Active Groups

	Sedentary (n = 53)	Active (n = 48)	
Characteristic	n%		χ^2
Race			
White	50 (94)	43 (90)	0.27
Nonwhite	3 (6)	5 (10)	
Marital status			
Married	51 (96)	44 (92)	6.28
Divorced	2 (4)	0 (0)	
Single	0 (0)	4 (8)	
Educational level			
High school	8 (15)	6 (12)	12.64*
Some college	19 (36)	11 (23)	
BA/BS	21 (40)	13 (27)	
Postbachelor	5 (9)	18 (38)	
Cesarean birth	17 (32)	12 (25)	0.62
	Mean (± *SD*)		
Age (years)	27.2 (3.8)	28.4 (4.1)	1.57

* $p < 0.01$

Note. From "Pregnancy outcomes among active and sedentary primiparous women," by P. Horns et al., 1996, *Journal of Obstetric, Gynecologic and Neonatal Nursing, 25*(1,) p. 51.

were found between the sedentary and the active groups on mean time of stage-1 labor, stage-2 labor, total time of labor, or the newborns' Apgar scores at 1 minute. Although all Apgar scores were above 7.0, the mean Apgar score at 5 minutes was significantly higher for the newborns of the women in the sedentary group.

Another statistical procedures used to test the difference between group means is ANOVA. Whereas the *t*-test is used to compare the means between two groups, ANOVA compares the means of two or more groups. The results of calculations for ANOVA are expressed as an F ratio that compares the variance between groups to the variance within groups.

Correlation procedures used to describe relationships between and among variables were mentioned earlier in this chapter. The Pearson *r* is a widely used correlation coefficient for describing the relationship between two variables, each measured on an interval or ratio scale. Sometimes correlations between several variables are displayed in a correlation matrix. In Table 8.7, the correlation matrix from the Budin

TABLE 8.6 Example of *t*-test Results. Means, Standard Deviations and *t*-tests Comparing Sedentary and Active Women on Selected Pregnancy Outcome Variables

Variable	Sedentary		Active		*t*-test
	Mean (± *SD*)				
Total sample *n* =	53		48		
Weight gain (lbs)	38.2	(12.9)	35.9	(11.6)	0.91
Birth weight	3464	(434)	2496	(486)	0.33
Gestational age (weeks)	39.2	(4.3)	39.9	(1.4)	1.08
Number of discomforts	8.7	(2.3)	7.5	(3.0)	2.11
Apgar 1 minute	8.1	(1.3)	7.9	(1.1)	0.59
Apgar 5 minutes	9.1	(0.5)	8.8	(0.7)	2.24
Vaginal delivery *n* =	36		36		
Stage 1 labor (hours)	12.6	(10.3)	11.5	(5.8)	0.51
Stage 2 labor (hours)	2.2	(4.2)	2.0	(3.1)	0.58
Total labor (hours)	14.6	(10.6)	13.4	(6.6)	0.60
Apgar 1 minute	8.4	(0.6)	8.0	(1.1)	1.79
Apgar 5 minute	9.2	(0.4)	8.8	(0.6)	2.96*
Cesarean delivery *n* =	17		12		
Apgar 1 minute	7.4	(1.9)	7.6	(1.2)	0.36
Apgar 5 minute	8.6	(0.7)	8.7	(0.9)	0.52

* $p < 0.01$

Note. From "Pregnancy outcomes among active and sedentary primiparous women," by P. Horns et al., 1996, *Journal of Obstetric, Gynecologic and Neonatal Nursing, 25*(1), p. 53.

(1998, p. 61) study shows the correlations among the variables: primary treatment alternatives, symptom distress, social support, and psychosocial adjustment to breast cancer in unmarried women. Notice that the asterisks (*) indicate statistically significant relationships.

An advanced statistical procedure used to express a relationship among several independent variables and one dependent variable is multiple regression. Multiple regression, expressed by the R-square statistic, is used to explain the amount of variance in a dependent variable contributed by each of the independent variables, collectively or independently. Table 8.8 (Budin, 1998, p. 161) shows the summary statistics for a multiple regression analysis used in the previously mentioned study. In this case the variables of primary treatment alternatives, symptom distress, and social support accounted for 57% of the variance in psychosocial adjustment.

In addition to the statistical procedures mentioned in this chapter, there are many others, including advanced or multivariate statistics procedures. Detailed explanation of how these and other tests are calculated, and when one is used rather than another, is beyond the

TABLE 8.7 An Example of a Correlation Matrix. Zero-Order Intercorrelations of the Main Study Variables

Variable	1	2	3	4
1. Primary Treatment Alternatives	—	−0.12	−0.09	−0.12
2. Perceived Social Support		—	−0.22*	−0.29**
3. Symptom Distress			—	0.74**
4. Psychosocial Adjustment to Breast Cancer				—

* $p < 0.05$, two-tailed; ** $p < 0.01$, two-tailed.
Note. From "Psychosocial adjustment to breast cancer in unmarried women," by W. Budin, 1998, *Research in Nursing and Health, 21,* p. 161.

purpose of this book, and again you are referred to a basic text on statistics. Two excellent books are *Statistical Methods for Health Care Research* (Munro, 1997) and *Data Analysis and Statistics for Nursing Research* (Polit-O'Hara, 1996). For a précis, and terse and to the point reference, read Duffy (1988).

Remember that the purpose of statistical analysis is to make possible the interpretation of collected data; it does not correct data that happen to be biased or that are based on inadequate or inappropriate samples. Moreover, nursing data that have been found to be highly significant statistically also need to be examined in terms of their clinical significance; that is, whether the findings are of any value to nursing.

SUMMARY

As a result of inspecting, organizing, and displaying the data in as many ways as appropriate and subjecting the data to statistical analysis when

TABLE 8.8 Example of Multiple Regression. Multiple Regression of Primary Treatment Alternatives, Perceived Social Support, and Symptom Distress on Psychosocial Adjustment to Breast Cancer ($n = 101$)

Variable entered	Beta	R	R^2	R^2 Change	$F(3,7)$ Change
Primary Treatment Alternatives	−0.071				
Perceived Social Support	−0.142				
Symptom Distress	0.702	0.754	0.569	0.569	42.75*

* $p < 0.001$.
Note. From "Psychosocial adjustment to breast cancer in unmarried women," by W. Budin, 1998, *Research in Nursing and Health, 21,* p. 161.

indicated, the researcher is able to formulate a statement of findings. Now it is time to interpret the findings draw conclusions, and consider the implications of these findings and make recommendations.

REFERENCES

American Psychological Association. (1994). *Publication manual of the American Psychological Association* (4th ed.). Washington, DC: Author.

Beck, C. (1992). The lived experience of postpartum depression: A phenomenological study. *Nursing Research, 41,* 166–170.

Budin, W. (1998). Psychosocial adjustment to breast cancer in unmarried women. *Research in Nursing and Health, 21,* 155–166.

Cusson, R., Madonia, J., & Taekman, J. (1997). The effect of environment on body site temperature in full-term neonates. *Nursing Research, 46*(4), 202–207.

Duffy, M. E. (1988). Statistics: Friend or foe? *Nursing and Health Care, 9,* 73–75.

Hansell, P., Hughes, C., Caliandro, G., Russo, P., Budin, W., Hartman, B., & Hernandez, O. (1998). The effects of a social support boosting intervention on stress, coping, and social support in caregivers of children with HIV/AIDS. *Nursing Research, 47*(2), 79–86.

Horns, P., Ratcliffe, L., Leggett, J., & Swanson, M. (1996). Pregnancy outcomes among active and sedentary primiparous women. *Journal of Obstetric, Gynecologic and Neonatal Nursing, 25*(1), 49–54.

Keefe, M. R. (1987). Comparison of neonatal nighttime sleep-wake patterns in nursery versus rooming-in environments. *Nursing Research, 36,* 140–144.

Munro, B. (1997). *Statistical methods for health care research* (3rd ed.). Philadelphia: Lippincott.

Pettengill, M., Gillies, D., & Clark, C. (1994). Factors encouraging and discouraging use of nursing research findings. *Image: Journal of Nursing Scholarship, 26,* 143–147.

Polit-O'Hara, D. (1996). *Data analysis and statistics for nursing research.* Stamford, CT: Appleton & Lange.

Rentschler, D. D. (1991). Correlates of successful breastfeeding. *Image: Journal of Nursing Scholarship, 23,* 151–154.

Schroeder, C. (1996). Women's experience of bed rest in high-risk pregnancy. *Image, 28,* 253–258.

Trossman, S. (1998). Nursing profession must mirror society's diversity. *American Nurse, 30*(1), 25.

9

Discussion of Findings, Conclusions, and Recommendations

Perhaps the admonition "be cautious" is the best advice that can be given to the beginning researcher who, having analyzed the data, has reached the point of discussing findings, drawing some conclusions, and making some recommendations. Although it is important for the investigator to point out and discuss some of the possible meanings of the findings as shown by the data, it is equally important that you avoid drawing conclusions that go beyond those indicated by the data and making recommendations that cannot be justified by the results of the study.

SOME EXAMPLES OF DISCUSSION, CONCLUSIONS, AND RECOMMENDATIONS

In the study of adolescents' perceptions of pain during labor, Sittner, Hudson, Grossman, and Gaston-Johansson (1998) illustrate how one can discuss study findings in terms of limitations involved and yet make suggestions about nursing care that are based on the findings. The authors point out that the small sample size and its racial homogeneity limit the generalization of these findings to other pregnant adolescents. They also discuss the failure of the labor and delivery nurses to collect data throughout all the participant's three labor phases. They suggest that future research involving a larger random sample of heterogeneous participants at all three labor phases might clarify pregnant adolescents' experiences of pain during the progression of labor. In view of these limitations, Sittner et al. suggest that the results of this study may still provide nurses with a greater understanding of the intensity and quality of pain adolescents experience during the progression of labor. These findings may assist nurses in individualizing nursing care and implementing pain-relieving interventions.

In the intervention study to test the effect of a social support boosting intervention on stress, coping, and social support in caregivers of children with HIV/AIDS, the authors caution,

> The results of this study need to be understood within the context of the study's limitations. The caregivers who participated in this study were a highly challenging group of individuals, encountering stressors that were numerous, complex, and erratic. Because of the unpredictable course of HIV/AIDS, maintaining a sample over time was extremely difficult. (Hansell et al., 1998, p. 85)

In the Rentschler (1991) study "Correlates of successful breast-feeding," the author noted that the success rate (70% of the mothers successfully breast-fed for 6 weeks) was higher in comparison with that reported by the national surveys (which at the time was 60%). Rentschler suggested that the higher success rate was most likely related to demographic characteristics of the sample. The participants were generally well-educated, relatively affluent, and likely to hold administrative or professional positions. She related this to the literature, which indicated that social class and education are positively related to the decision to breast-feed. Beyond the effect homogeneity of the sample may have had on the results of the study, she concluded that the findings supported the premise that women who are knowledgeable about breast-feeding and are high achievers will be successful at breast-feeding.

You might find it profitable to look at the "findings" and "discussion" sections of other study reports, noting especially the use of such phrases as "results seem to indicate," "this finding suggests," and "possible explanations are," which reflect investigators' caution in reporting. Also note how the investigators relate findings to the purpose of the study, its theoretical rationale, and the hypotheses made before the study began. It is all right to start reading a research study's ending first; the thrill is in the research, not the mystery!

LIMITATIONS

Important limitations should always be recognized in the published report of any study. They may simply be implied, or they may be spelled out early in the report and repeated in the discussion of the findings. Budin (1998) carefully pointed out limitations to the method of sample selection used in her study:

> The internal validity of this study may have been influenced by the process through which individuals were approached and asked to volunteer to participate. Although the response rate was excellent (88%) for the individuals who agreed to participate, the question of selection bias must be raised. Perhaps only highly motivated women were interested in participating. It may be that those who refused to participate were those who were more symptomatic and distressed by their illness experience than those who agreed to participate. (p. 164)

Budin also acknowledges a somewhat homogeneous group in education and socioeconomic status. She cautions that the results of this study cannot be generalized beyond this population of unmarried women.

In the report of the study by Trice (1990), the author also noted limitations to the study that precluded generalization. The sample was made up entirely of Whites, and most participants were female. His suggestions for future research included repeating the study on different ethnic groups, different age groups, and perhaps another group of elderly Whites consisting mostly of men.

Redeker, Mason, Wykpisz, and Glica (1996) identified the limitations of their study. They point out that medications, such as narcotic analgesics, hypnotics, sedatives, and cardiovascular drugs, that are routinely administered to CABG patients are known to influence sleep patterns. The medications administered to the current sample were too varied in type and timing to permit examination of their impact. They suggest that the relationships between sleep and commonly used postoperative drugs should be considered in future studies. Although the investigator may not be able to control all the variables that may influence the results, it is essential that potential confounding variables and limitations be recognized and discussed.

The most common limitations in clinical nursing studies are (1) small sample size and unrepresentativeness of the sample, for example, a small convenience sample in one or two hospitals, and (2) the use of relatively untested tools for gathering data, for example, schedules or questionnaires that the investigator developed for a study but that were not adequately tested for validity and reliability. Sherman (1996) acknowledged the low reliability of the Templer Death Anxiety Scale in her study and recommended further testing of this instrument. She also speculated that the low reliability may have been related to the forced true or false response format, which limited the response possibilities for each question. It was suggested that a Likert response format, which offers a broader range of responses, may allow a researcher to better detect the real feelings of an individual. In their review of Trice (1990), Feldman and Hott (1991) raise the question about limitations in Trice's study because the participants, mostly female elderly Whites (2 men and 9 women), are not representative of the general population. This does not mean, however, that the nurse cannot learn from an assessment of the clients' meaningful life experience. This is not meant to suggest that small clinical studies should not be done but only that the limitations should be explicitly recognized. In fact, one outcome of small studies may be ideas and hypotheses for larger, more sophisticated studies.

RELATING CONCLUSIONS TO THE PURPOSE OF THE STUDY

It is very important for the investigator to remember that the conclusions reached in a study must be related to the purpose, hypothesis, and results of the data analysis. For example, Sherman (1996), whose study used Rogers' framework of the science of unitary human beings to examine relationships among spirituality, perceived social support, death anxiety, and nurses' willingness to care for AIDS patients, stated in her discussion that "statistical support of the three hypotheses provided preliminary validity for the propositions derived from both the science of unitary human beings and the literature." Budin (1998) summarizes her conclusion as follows:

> The results support the hypothesized relations among symptom distress, perceived social support, and psychosocial adjustment to breast cancer in unmarried women. Symptom distress emerged as the variable accounting for the most variance in psychosocial adjustment. Primary treatment alternatives did not correlate with any of the study variables. For the most part, the unmarried women is this sample were experiencing relatively low levels of problems with adjustment during the late postoperative recovery phase and perceived moderately high levels of social support from individuals identified in their support networks. (p. 162)

Budin then goes on to discuss each of the findings in terms of the related literature and how the findings from this study either support or conflict with findings from previous research. The discussion section builds a case for why this study is important and how it adds to the body of knowledge on adjustment to breast cancer.

A look at other studies mentioned in this chapter (Hansell et al., 1998; Redeker et al., 1996; Rentschler, 1991; Trice, 1990; Sherman, 1996; Sittner et al., 1998) will show that the investigators' discussion, conclusions, and recommendations were consistent with the stated purpose or hypotheses of the studies as well as with the method of study and the findings. For example, the purpose in the Rentschler study was to gain a better understanding of the relationship of a pregnant woman's motivation to breast-feed and her knowledge about breast-feeding to success in breast-feeding (Rentschler, 1991, p. 151). The method used to collect data was descriptive. Rentschler administered prenatal questionnaire instruments that assessed personal data, achievement motivation, and knowledge about breast-feeding and another questionnaire about the breast-feeding experience 6 weeks post partum. Her findings, conclusions, and recommendations appear to be consistent with the purposes and data analysis.

SERENDIPITOUS FINDINGS

No discussion of findings would be complete without at least a brief mention of the role of serendipity in research. One occasionally hears of valuable findings that appear to occur spontaneously while the investigator is carrying out a study related to something else. In exploring the breast-feeding experiences of women, Lothian (1995) found that the baby's own characteristics and capabilities influenced the process of breast-feeding in unexpected ways and, over time, emerged as the most important factors influencing baby satisfaction and ultimately breast-feeding duration. She concluded that, if "it takes two to breast-feed," it is not enough for the mother to be committed to breast-feeding, have knowledge of the mechanics of breast-feeding, and be supported in her efforts to be successful. It is essential that breast-feeding women and providers of breast-feeding education and support be aware of the critical role that babies play in breast-feeding. The trained, experienced observer is likely to recognize a serendipitous finding when it presents itself, but the novice may pass it over. The moral is that if something in the study keeps "bugging" you, take time out to examine it. You may have found another study in the making, or you may have made a discovery more important than any inherent in the purpose of your study.

SUMMARY

In concluding this chapter, we suggest that you review the findings, conclusions, and recommendations of other studies in the literature. Look particularly to see whether they are consistent with the purpose, theoretical rationale, hypothesis, method of collecting data, and analysis of the data. Note also whether limitations of the study are recognized and taken into account in the conclusions reached.

REFERENCES

Budin, W. (1998). Psychosocial adjustment to breast cancer in unmarried women. *Research in Nursing and Health, 21,* 155–166.

Feldman, H. R., & Hott, J. R. (1991). Light up your practice with nursing research. *Journal of the New York State Nurses Association, 22,* 2–11.

Hansell, P., Hughes, C., Caliandro, G., Russo, P., Budin, W., Hartman, B., & Hernandez, O. (1998). The effects of a social support boosting intervention on stress, coping, and social support in caregivers of children with HIV/AIDS. *Nursing Research, 47*(2), 79–86.

Lothian, J. (1995). It takes two to breastfeed: The baby's role in successful breastfeeding. *Journal of Nurse-Midwifery, 40,* 328–334.

Redeker, N., Mason, D., Wykpisz, E., & Glica, B. (1996). Sleep patterns in women after coronary artery bypass surgery. *Applied Nursing Research, 9*(3), 115–122.

Rentschler, D. D. (1991). Correlates of successful breastfeeding. *Image: Journal of Nursing Scholarship, 23,* 151–154.

Sherman, D. (1996). Nurses' willingness to care for AIDS patients and spirituality, social support, and death anxiety. *Image, 28,* 205–213.

Sittner, B., Hudson, D., Grossman, C., & Gaston-Johansson, F. (1998). Adolescents' perceptions of pain during labor. *Clinical Nursing Research, 7*(1), 82–93.

Trice, L. B. (1990). Meaningful life experience in the elderly. *Image: Journal of Nursing Scholarship, 22,* 248–251.

10

Use of Computers in Nursing Research

The use of computers and the explosion of information technology has become an integral part of nursing research. Computers are an invaluable tool for researchers and consumers of research because of their speed, accuracy, and flexibility. A major task for all professional nurses is to process and integrate information so that it becomes useful knowledge—knowledge that can guide clinical practice. Nurses must be aware of and have easy access to the information available. Moreover, nurses need to be able to analyze, synthesize, and integrate this information into a knowledge base (Sills, 1997). Billings (1996) describes how information technology helps to keep nursing knowledge accessible by establishing vehicles for communicating nursing knowledge and building links among clinicians, researchers, and educators. Computer applications that support the research process are numerous. In this chapter we will identify and describe some of the more common applications of computers for nursing research.

COMPUTERIZED LITERATURE SEARCHES

Computers are particularly useful for accessing the large electronic databases available for conducting a literature search (see chapter 4). In fact, computerized literature searches are now considered commonplace. The Interagency Council on Information Resources for Nursing (ICIRN) (1996) listed 26 computerized databases of interest to nurses and other health care providers. The database of most importance to consumers of nursing research is the CINAHL. This database provides authoritative coverage of the professional literature in nursing and 17 allied health disciplines, biomedicine, consumer health, and health science librarianship. Virtually all nursing journals are indexed, along with publications from the ANA and the NLN. CINAHL also provides access to health care books, book chapters, pamphlets, nursing dissertations, selected conference proceedings, audiovisual material, and educational software (Cumulative Index to Nursing and Allied Health Literature [CINAHL], 1998).

Sigma Theta Tau's Virginia Henderson International Nursing Library also offers electronic services that can be tapped into from home and university offices. This "unique, state-of-the-art computerized facility provides access to current nursing research and the opportunity to network globally with nurses and health care professionals" (Sigma Theta Tau International, 1998c). The Registry of Nursing Research, also available online through the Virginia Henderson Library, contains biographical data about nurse researchers, their research programs and studies, and results of their studies, including abstracts and information about related studies (Sigma Theta Tau International, 1998a). A growing number of nursing journals are now available online that allow you to browse the table of contents for articles of interest. Some online journals require subscriptions and provide full-length articles as well as abstracts. The *Online Journal of Knowledge Synthesis for Nursing* is a peer reviewed electronic journal that provides critical reviews of research pertinent to clinical practice and research situations (Sigma Theta Tau International, 1998b). Electronic databases used for literature searches in medicine, biology, sociology, psychology, or education, may also be useful. Examples include MEDLINE (1998), Psychological Abstracts (PsychLIT), and Educational Resources Information Center (ERIC) (Sinclair, 1997).

Most university libraries can provide individuals with access to search these electronic databases. Many databases are also available on CD-ROM or can be accessed from home on personal computers with Internet connections. Once you have narrowed down your topic and identified a few key words, your search will provide a computer-generated list of citations pertinent to the selected topic. Some computerized searches will provide abstracts of the articles in addition to the citation. Computerized literature searches are rapid, convenient, and cost effective. For excellent references on keeping abreast of the literature electronically, see Nicoll (1998) and Sinclair (1997).

DATABASES FOR ACCESSING MEASUREMENT TOOLS

Computerized databases are also useful for locating instruments for data collection (see chapter 7). For example, "The Health and Psychological Instruments Online" (HaPI, 1998) provides information on questionnaires, rating scales, interview forms, checklists, vignettes or scenarios, indexes, coding schemes or manuals, projective techniques, and tests. Information is abstracted from leading journals covering the health and psychosocial sciences. The Buros Institute of Mental Measurements (1998), also available online, publishes the *Mental Measurements Yearbook* and *Tests in Print* series.

OTHER COMPUTERIZED SOURCES FOR GATHERING DATA

In addition to accessing information about relevant literature and instruments by computer, nurse researchers can use the computer for data collection and retrieval (Goldsmith, 1996). Computers not only assist nurses in monitoring and regulating patient's vital processes, planning, and recording patient care but also are invaluable in information retrieval in the data collection phase of the research process. Computer technology allows for interface of biophysiological instruments and computers (Harrison, 1989). Collection of varied simultaneous clinical data at the bedside provides the nurse researcher with resources that were never available so rapidly before and is only limited by the clinician's creativity in their application. For example, Redeker, Mason, Wykpisz, and Glica (1996) describe the use of a wrist-worn computerized actigraph to record sleep patterns in women post CABG surgery, and Keefe (1987) used computerized monitors to measure sleep-wake cycles in newborns.

There are many informational and statistical databases from government agency websites and others to provide research data (see appendix E). The U.S. Department of Health and Human Services provides information about biomedical research, health services research, and health statistics. The National Center for Health Statistics provides links to a variety of sites for health statistics, including AIDS/HIV information; aging, elderly care; alcohol and drug information; cancer information; cardiovascular disease and risk factors; child health; and women's health. Kovner (1989) provides examples of computerized databases for nursing research and quality assurance, discussing their pros and cons, and gives examples of both bibliographic and actual databases. Kovner suggests that the use of computerized data shortens data collection and data entry, speeding up knowledge acquisition to improve patient care.

Data collection from survey questionnaires that require research participants to mark their responses on Likert-type scales, semantic differentials, and dichotomous responses categories can also be simplified through the use of computer technology. An optical scanner attached to a microcomputer can markedly facilitate the collection and management of self-report research data. Dennis (1994) describes the construction of scannable questionnaire forms, highlights the capabilities of the optical scanner, outlines the scanning procedure, and discusses the management of derived data sets. Her experience using scannable questionnaire forms in numerous research projects over the course of several years demonstrated that participants were receptive to this form of data collection and had no more difficulty with it than might be encountered with questionnaires in a manual format. The cost, however, of acquiring the optical scanner hardware and software is a consideration for the researcher with limited funds.

DATA MANAGEMENT AND STATISTICAL ANALYSIS FOR QUANTITATIVE RESEARCH

Computers have revolutionized quantitative research methods by making possible the kinds of operations that could not have been attempted previously. In the past, data analysis was a tedious process done by hand. High-speed computers take the tedium out of statistical computations, allowing the calculation of complex statistical procedures in a brief period of time. The ability of the computer to perform these calculations quickly and accurately allows a researcher to spend time searching for patterns in the data and answering questions of interest, rather than on the mechanics of computation (Enspruch, 1998).

Statistical software packages are indispensable for organizing, managing, and analyzing quantitative data. The packages most widely used by nurse researchers include the Statistical Package for the Social Sciences (SPSS), Biomedical Programs (BMDP), and Statistical Analysis System (SAS). Each contains programs to handle a variety of procedures for data management and statistical analyses. Researchers using these packaged programs do not need to know computer programming. They are designed to be easy to use by individuals with minimal or no computer skills. A number of books and tutorials are available that introduce users to some computer terminology, demonstrate that sophisticated skills are not needed to use the computer, and explain the steps required to prepare data for computer analysis. (Enspruch, 1998; Hedderson & Fisher, 1993).

Before entering quantitative data into the computer, the data must be organized and coded. A codebook allows the researcher to identify each variable in a study and assign an abbreviated nickname to the variable (Lebo, 1993). It also allows the researcher to assign descriptive labels to the numerical codes that are entered into the computer. Data entry into the computer is a very important part of the research process. It must be done carefully and attentively. Careful data entry will reduce the amount of time needed to clean the data (check for errors) once analyses have begun. Although computers can provide speed and accuracy in statistical analyses, one must be aware that the "output" is only as good as the "input." As the saying goes, "garbage in, garbage out." Using the computer for statistical analysis can be tedious, time consuming, frustrating and, if not carefully monitored, fraught with errors. Developing a codebook, coding the raw data onto a computer entry form, and then entering the data through numerous key strokes takes patience, accuracy, and time. Users must also have a basic knowledge of statistics and be able to communicate to the computer information about the variables and how the data are to be analyzed.

COMPUTERS AND QUALITATIVE RESEARCH

The use of computer technology has also emerged as a significant component in qualitative research methodology (Anderson, 1987; Kelly & Sime, 1990; Pilkington, 1996; Taft, 1993). Computer-assisted data analysis is the latest in a series of technological advances that have transformed qualitative research. Qualitative data analysis is labor intensive and incorporates both mechanical and interpretative functions. In the past, analysis of qualitative data required hours and hours of cutting and pasting pages and pages of narrative material (Morse & Morse, 1989). Schroeder (1996) described how interview transcripts of women experiencing bed rest in high-risk pregnancies were entered into a computer data management program and codes that seemed to capture the pattern of the interview were defined and entered. The computer program was used to sort and retrieve coded segments that were then filed both individually by woman and according to code. Segments were reread to see if they actually fit the code word assigned and, if not, moved to the appropriate code file. Computer programs save time and increase the efficiency of the mechanical tasks of data management. Because of the continuous interplay between data management and data interpretation, however, the use of computers in qualitative analysis may influence conceptual as well as mechanical activities (Taft, 1993; Tesch, 1991). Although computer programs facilitate the management and reorganization of data and prepare data for interpretation, they cannot replace the thinking and decision making that are the heart of qualitative analysis. The burden of interpretation rests on the researcher. Computer enhancements that build connections between categories of data may suggest relationships between concepts, but it is up to the researcher to establish the meaning and significance of suggested relationships through intensive analysis. Among the most widely used programs developed specifically for analyzing qualitative data are QUALPRO, HyperQual, and Ethnograph (Taft, 1993; Tesch, 1991; Weitzman & Miles, 1995).

THE INTERNET AS TOOL FOR NURSING RESEARCH

Millions of people have discovered the riches of the Internet and have joined the swelling numbers of cyberspace explorers (Bauman, 1997). The Internet, a global network of interconnected local and regional computer networks, offers instant access to information worldwide (Hubbard & Thurn, 1997). A key factor in the Internet's evolution has been the development of the World Wide Web (WWW), a hypertext system that provides an intuitive "point and click" interface to data on the Internet. When the computer mouse clicks on a hypertext link, the user is taken to another website or another page within the website. To navigate the Web you need a program called a Web browser, such as Netscape Navigator or Microsoft Internet Explorer. New Web sites are appearing daily. Lybecker (1998) notes the sheer quantity of information on the Internet can be daunting, especially since there is no central directory. She compares it to going to the library and finding that the books are in no particular order and that there is no card catalog. Search engines such as Yahoo (www.yahoo.com), AltaVista (www.altavista.digital.com), and Lycos (www.lycos.com) can help to organize your search of the Internet. By typing in a few key words or "strings of text" you will be provided with a list of many useful (and not so useful) sites that match your search terms. Sorting through these sites can be extremely time consuming, however. Each Web site has a specific address or Uniform Resource Locator (URL) consisting of a string of characters that usually describes the site. Using bookmarks is an excellent way to keep track of your favorite Web pages without having to remember their addresses. A bookmark comprises the title of the Web page and the URL. When you have located a Web site of interest you can save the location with a bookmark.

There is a staggering amount of information available and accessible on the WWW. The sheer quantity of information can sometimes make it difficult to locate the best sites for one's needs. The remainder of this section will point out some of the more useful sites for obtaining information related to nursing research from the Internet (see Nicoll, 1998, for a comprehensive guide).

The Internet is an excellent tool for finding information about available research grants from both public and private sectors. Some institutions even provide their application forms on the Internet. The Community of Science provides access to a database providing funding information from federal and state governments, foundations, professional societies, associations, corporations, and other scientific organizations. Other useful funding sources with Web sites include the Agency for Health Care Policy and Research, the Robert Wood Johnson Foundation, the NIH, the NINR, and Sigma Theta Tau International (see appendix E for Internet addresses).

In addition to information retrieval, the Internet is an important resource for communication. The Internet is connecting individuals in a way no other technology has been able. Electronic mail (e-mail), touted by some as the most effective method of communication, is one of the main uses of the Internet. For many, e-mail is preferred over phone calls or traditional mail and is used for many purposes (Hutchinson, 1997).

The need for one user to communicate via e-mail with many users gave rise to modified e-mail applications, including mailing lists, Listserves, and newsgroups. A mailing list is a list of e-mail addresses used to forward messages to groups of people. Listserves are electronic mailing lists. Subscribing to the list enables you to send an e-mail message to the entire list of subscribers. Messages sent by other subscribers go to you and everyone else on the list. The effect is that of the discussion group held via e-mail. Generally, a mailing list is used to discuss a particular set of topics. There are Listserves or discussion groups available for sharing and exchanging information on just about any topic imaginable. For example NURSERES is a Listserve that provides discussion on nursing research and related health and professional issues. To subscribe to this Listserve, simply send an e-mail message to listserv@kentvm.kent.edu, then in the body of the message type "Subscribe NURSERES Firstname Lastname" (where "Firstname" is your first name and "Lastname" is your last name). Be warned. When you join a mailing list, you will receive lots of e-mail. When you join a Listserve you will receive instructions on how to discontinue your subscription. Be sure you save these instructions (see appendix E for other Listserves).

A more recent application that uses technology called Internet Relay Chat (IRC) allows for "real-time" communication in which messages that are typed appear instantly on another's computer screen. "Chat rooms" and many discussion groups use this technology. Nicoll (1998) provides a complete list of chat rooms and discussion groups.

Brennan, Moore, and Smyth (1995) described the effects of a computer network that was specially designed to provide information, communication, and decision-support functions for caregivers of persons with Alzheimer Disease (see chapter 7). There are a growing number of online support groups available for a variety of health-related conditions (Hutchinson, 1996). Wood and Delozier (1997) provide a comprehensive reference devoted entirely to cancer resources on the Internet.

Computer networks can also be used as a way to access and recruit participants for a research study. Wilmoth (1995) describes a creative approach in which she posted a message on the Cancer Support Group Bulletin Board and received 11 replies within 24 hours. Several respondents also participated in a breast cancer support group and offered to distribute copies of the questionnaire to support group members. This method contributed 4% of the sample in an inexpensive and timely way. Although using computer networks to access a sample has tremendous potential, one must exercise caution when using this approach because it is hard to validate the trustworthiness of the responses or the respondents. The issue of selection bias must also be considered.

Another example of an innovative website designed to promote information sharing in health care by nurses, physicians, and other health care professionals is the Best Practice Network (1998). This Web site facilitates the exchange of ideas, encourages collaboration in results-oriented problem solving, and enables health care professionals to learn from one another the best in current practices that will promote excellence in patient care and community well-being. For example, within the Best Practice Network, an interdisciplinary team was convened to assess the current status of skin care, to search literature and contact skin experts, to analyze alternatives, and to design a program and implement it.

SUMMARY

In this chapter we have discussed a variety of computer applications useful to nurse researchers and consumers of research. The computer is an indispensable tool for accessing the large electronic databases available for conducting a literature search, finding instruments, locating sources for funding, or finding other information. Computers are also useful for data collection, data management, and data analysis in both quantitative and qualitative studies. The Internet has limitless potential as a source for information retrieval and as a tool to enhance communication among researchers and others. As we move into the new millennium, our scientific knowledge and understanding can be enhanced by the continued use of computers and information technology as a tool for nursing research.

REFERENCES

Anderson, N. (1987). Computer applications for qualitative analysis. *Western Journal of Nursing Research*, *9*(3), 408–411.

Bauman, A. (1997). APNs tap vast Internet Resources. *Spectrum: Greater New York Metro Edition, 9*(19), 8.

Best Practice Network. (1998, February 20). *About the Best Practice Network* [Online]. Available: http://best4health.org/html/hist.htm

Billings, D. (1996). From colored pens to computers. *Reflections, 2nd Quarter, 23*(2).

Biomedical Programs (BMDP). Statistical Software, Inc., Suite 316, 1440 Sepulveda Blvd., Los Angeles, CA 90025.

Brennan, P., Moore, S., & Smyth, K. (1995). The effects of a special computer network on caregivers of persons with Alzheimer's disease. *Nursing Research, 44*(3), 166–172.

Buros, O. (1998, February 18). *Buros Institute for mental measurements.* [Online]. Available: http://www.unl.edu/buros/ (.

Cumulative Index to Nursing and Allied Health Literature (CINAHL). (1998, January 14). *CINAHL Information Systems for Nursing and Allied Health* [On-line]. Available: http://www.cinahl.com

Dennis, K. (1994). Managing questionnaire data through optical scanning technology. *Nursing Research, 43*(6), 376–378.

Enspruch, E. (1998). *An Introductory Guide to SPSS for Windows.* Thousand Oaks, CA: Sage.

Goldsmith, J. (1996). Computers and nurses changing hospital care. *Reflections, 2nd Quarter, 23*(2), 8–10.

HaPI. (1998). *Health and psychosocial instruments.* Behavioral Measurements Database Service, P.O. Box 1100287, Pittsburgh, PA.

Harrison, L. (1989). Interfacing bioinstruments with computers for data collection in nursing research. *Research in Nursing and Health, 12*(2), 129–133.

Hedderson, J., & Fisher, M. (1993). *SPSS made simple.* Belmont, CA: Wadsworth.

Hubbard, S., & Thurn, A. (1997). National Cancer Institute's CancerNet: A reliable source of current cancer information on the Internet. In M. S. Wood & E. Delozier (Eds.), *Cancer resources on the Internet* (pp. 15–22). Binghamton, NY: Haworth Press.

Hutchinson, D. (1997). A nurse's guide to the Internet, *RN, 60*(1), 46–51.

Hutchinson, D. (1996). *An Internet guide for the health professional* (2nd ed.). Sacramento, CA: New Winds.

Institute for Natural Resources. (1996). *The Internet: A guide for health professionals.* Berkeley, CA: Institute for Natural Resources.

Interagency Council on Information Resources for Nursing. (1996). Essential nursing references, *Nurse Health Care Perspective Commission, 17,* 255–259.

Keefe, M. R. (1987). Comparison of neonatal nighttime sleep-wake patterns in nursery versus rooming-in environments. *Nursing Research, 36,* 140–144.

Kelly, A., & Sime, A. (1990). Language as research data: Application of computer content analysis in nursing research. *Advances in Nursing Science, 12*(3), 32–40.

Kovner, C. (1989). Using computerized databases for nursing research and quality assurance. *Computers in Nursing, 7,* 228–231.

Lebo, M. (1993). Code books—A critical link in the research process. *Western Journal of Nursing Research 15,* 377–385.

Lybecker, C. (1998). Surfing the net. *Maternal Child Nursing, 23*(1), 17–21.

MEDLINE. (1998, January 14). *Free Medline: PubMed and Internet Grateful Med* [On-line]. Available: http://www.nlm.nih.gov/databases/freemedl.html

Morse, J., & Morse, R. (1989). QUAL: A mainframe program for qualitative data analysis. *Nursing Research, 38*(3), 188–189.

National Center for Health Statistics. (1998). [On-line]. Available: http://www.cdc.gov/nchswww/index/htm

Nicoll, L. (1998). *Nurses guide to the Internet* (2nd ed.). Philadelphia: Lippincott.

Pilkington, F. (1996). The use of computers in qualitative research. *Nursing Science Quarterly, 9*, 5–7.

Redeker, N., Mason, D., Wykpisz, E., & Glica, B. (1996). Sleep patterns in women after coronary artery bypass surgery. *Applied Nursing Research, 9*, 115–122.

Schroeder, C. (1996). Women's experience of bed rest in high-risk pregnancy. *Image, 28*(3), 253–258.

Sigma Theta Tau International. (1998a, January 14). *About Sigma Theta Tau International Registry of Nursing Research* [On-line]. Available: http://www.stti.iupui.edu/rnr/

Sigma Theta Tau International (1998b, January 14). *STTI Publications: Online journal of knowledge synthesis for nursing* [On-line]. Available: http://www.stti.iupui.edu/publications/journal/

Sigma Theta Tau International (1998c, January 14). *Virginia Henderson International Library* [On-line]. Available: http://www.stti.iupui.edu/library

Sills, G. (1997). The information age [Editorial]. *Journal of Psychiatric Nurses Association, 3*(3), 67.

Sinclair, V. (1987). Literature searches by computer. *Image, 19*, 35–37.

Statistical Analysis System (SAS). SAS Institute, Inc., SAS Campus Drive, Cary, NC, 27513-2414.

Statistical Package for the Social Sciences (SPSS). SPSS Inc., 233 Wacker Drive, Chicago, IL 60606-6507.

Taft, L. (1993). Computer-assisted qualitative research. *Research in Nursing and Health, 16*(5), 379–384.

Tesch, R. (1991). Computer programs that assist in the analysis of qualitative data: An overview. *Qualitative Health Research, 1*, 309–325.

U.S. Department of Health and Human Services. (1998). [On-line]. Available: www.os.dhhs.gov.

Weitzman, E., & Miles, M. (1995). *A software sourcebook: Computer programs for qualitative data analysis.* Thousand Oaks, CA: Sage.

Wilmoth, M. (1995). Computer networks as a source of research subjects. *Western Journal of Nursing Research, 17*, 335–338.

Wood, M. S., & Delozier, E. (Eds.). (1997). *Cancer resources on the Internet.* Binghamton, NY: Haworth Press.

11

The Research Report: Communicating the Findings

One task remains after a study is completed—the writing of the research report. When a study has been carried out meticulously and careful records have been kept as the study progressed, all material needed for the report is at hand. This will include a statement of the problem, the literature review that provided the documentation or scientific rationale and background for the study, the statement of questions to be examined or the hypotheses, the collected data, the data analysis, the conclusions that have been drawn, and further questions that have been raised.

Remember that the purpose of a research report is to communicate what was done in the study to the particular individuals interested in the topic of the study. Communication of nursing research must be carried out for two groups of people: other investigators and consumers of research. Other investigators need to be aware of your research as it relates to their own efforts; they may be interested in replicating your research or building on it and thus extending its value. Consumers of research need to know about your research if it is to make a difference in nursing practice. As Hinshaw (1989) points out, "One of the major challenges that continues to confront the profession is the ability to transfer research results into practice in a timely and effective manner" (p. 169). She describes this as a dilemma that nursing shares with other service professions and cites the complexity of communicating research findings, such as the multiple audiences for whom nursing results must be transferred and used, and making results available for nursing professionals as well as those upon whom our care is focused. These findings provide a way to legitimize professional nursing practice and to influence public policy. We know how significant this can be to determine funding for health care and nursing research.

A research report is intended to be informative, not entertaining. It should be well organized and written in a readable style using clear, simple language, however. Technical phrases and words should be used only when they are clearly needed. The following suggestions are intended for those who plan to write a research report but will also be helpful for consumers of research to gain a perspective of what goes into writing a report. Before starting to write, it is often helpful to consult references on writing, such as Sheridan and Dowdney (1997) or Barnum (1995). Barnum's primer for nurses is a step-by-step guide to developing professional writing skills and navigating the publication process. (See appendix A for a list of books on style and writing that may be helpful.) Those who are writing a report will also want to have a good, up-to-date dictionary and a thesaurus at hand while writing. If you use word processing software, know your tools. Is there a function to check spelling, to check grammar, or to provide synonyms? There are even software packages available to do bibliographic references. Check with resources at your local university or computer software store. There are electronic genies to work in your computer, but you must be their guide.

If you find it difficult to get started on writing your report, you are no different from many persons when they sit down to write (Beyerman, 1987; Corbett, 1987). There is only one way to handle this problem, however, and that is to put pencil to paper or to sit down at your keyboard. Hopefully, you will have discussed your ideas with a colleague, a research interest support group, or a mentor beforehand. Before you feel the "ecstasy" of doing research, relieve some of the "agony" by sharing it.

Since the organization of the report is very important in presenting your material well, you should probably start by making a tentative outline. The entries in the outline may very well become the various subheadings of your report. The next step is to compose the first paragraph of the first section. One way to start this paragraph is to make a simple statement of the problem studied. You may want to change this introduction later, but at the moment you need to get off the ground.

For the most part, research reports are written in the past tense. The authors cited in your literature review wrote in the past, your study was conducted in the past, and your study findings were also stated in the past. The present tense may be used, however, in reports and discussions of hypotheses and theories that are broadly accepted at the present time. The future tense is rarely used in research reports except for making recommendations or for extrapolating implications for nursing, when this is appropriate.

Reports should always be written objectively; that is, the personal pronoun "I" (or "we") should be reserved for the very rare occasions when writers need to refer to something specific about themselves. Otherwise, the term *investigator* is considered the correct one to use when referring to the person who conducted the research. The use of the passive voice may sometimes be necessary, but it can easily be overdone, to the extent that phrasing becomes awkward. Simply reporting what was done, in the active voice, should help to avoid this kind of awkwardness. It may be helpful for you to examine a few reports in the literature to see how other investigators have handled this aspect of their studies. You will find good as well as poor examples of writing; the former will help you know what to do, and the latter may point out what to avoid.

In your review of the literature always give credit to the authors of the material, whether paraphrased, quoted, or referred to and discussed. Remember that published material, whether in book or article form, is usually copyrighted. A major exception is government publications; these are in the public domain. Under Title 17 of the U.S. Code, part 302, paragraph (A), circular 91 (Revised March 1, 1991), works created after January 1, 1978, are protected by copyright during the author's lifetime and for 50 years after the author's death, after which the copyrighted material will go into public domain. (For information about this, contact the Superintendent of Documents, Washington, DC. Ask for Copyright Law of the United States of America, Circular 92, Purchase order #030-002-00170-5 or check at your library for #LC3.4/2:92.) Journals may allow the use of up to 500 words of copyrighted material without requiring permission, as long as it is properly cited. Policies about usage are usually stated in the front part of books (see the publisher's statement opposite the contents page in this book) and generally on the contents page or in a section on information for authors in journals.

When using quotations, check them carefully for accuracy and indicate the source in a footnote or in references at the end of the chapter or article. The books on writing in appendix A of this book offer suggestions on various approved ways of citing references. If you are submitting your research for publication, always check the journal and use the preferred format.

ORGANIZING THE REPORT

Unlike other forms of writing, scientific reports (with few exceptions) usually follow a rather standardized format. An outline for a nursing research report might look something like this:

Introduction
    Statement of the problem with a brief discussion of its significance

- Review of the literature pertinent to the problem studied
- Theoretical framework
- Hypotheses made or questions raised for study

Method
- Design for the study—detailed
- Study method
- Description of the sample and its delimitations
- Description of the instruments
- Description of the data analysis method

Findings
- Objective presentation of the summary of the data collected
- Tables, graphs, and other illustrations as needed
- Results of all tests of significance or other statistical measures

Discussion
- Conclusions
- Interpretation of findings
- Comparison of findings with those of other investigators, if pertinent
- Implications for nursing or recommendations for further study, or both

References
- All references cited in the report

Appendixes
- Copies of the instruments used (questionnaires, sample forms), letters of permission, protection of human subjects, and so on

The sections of the report should present objective, straightforward accounts of what was done in each step of the study. The opinions of the investigator have no place in a research report, with one exception. The investigator may wish to discuss the meaning of the findings or their implications for nursing and future research. Hickey (1990) provides a good example of this after a review of the literature about family needs in critical care. In such a case, the departure from the report and any statements based on the investigator's own interpretation of the data should be clearly indicated.

It is also important that the investigator relate the findings to both the purpose and the limitations of the study. For example, if the study sample was small, the significance of this should be recognized, or if the investigator did all the interviewing and recognized the existence of bias, this too should be pointed out. In the previous chapter a number of examples were provided on how authors describe the limitations of small sample size and nonrandom sample selection on the generalizability of their study. They make very specific recommendations for further research to deal with these design problems.

In the discussion of the data analysis and of the results of the study, it may be appropriate to include tables or graphs when these can show the data better, more clearly, or more dramatically than can be done by description in the text. Such "summary" tables assist in interpreting the data by displaying it in various ways. (Tables in chapter 8 present summarized data.) Unsummarized raw data (i.e., the actual tallies of data) belong in an appendix. Copies of instruments used (questionnaires, form letters, protection of human subjects, and so on) may also be included in an appendix.

If you are writing for a periodical or submitting your study for presentation at a research conference, you may be asked to prepare an abstract to accompany it. The abstract should be a very brief summary of the report and is usually limited to approximately 200 words. The abstract, although brief, should be informative. You should give the gist of the content of the article: a brief statement of the purpose of the study, the hypothesis, the methodology, and the results (see appendix C for guidelines on writing a research abstract). Some conference abstracts must be camera ready to be printed in conference proceedings. In addition, you may be asked to list key or index words that will facilitate electronic retrieval of your work. For example, in Hansell et al. (1998), key words are listed as social support, stress, coping, caregivers, and HIV/AIDS children. In Budin (1998) the key words are breast cancer, social support, psychosocial adjustment, symptom distress, and unmarried women.

Last, but by no means least, we should say a word about titles for reports. Titles of scientific reports should be simple, descriptive statements of the nature of the study. Cute or "breezy" titles are definitely out of place, not because they are catchy and therefore undignified but because other researchers searching the literature might not be able to tell from the title of your article whether it is of interest. For example, if you have made a study in which the attitudes of RN and social workers toward drug addicts were compared, the title of your report might well be "Comparison of the Attitudes of Registered Nurses and Social Workers Toward Drug Addicts." Hott (1980), however, was able to title her report appropriately and maintain a sense of "double entendre" in her study, "Best Laid Plans . . . Pre- and Postpartum Comparison of Self and Spouse in Primiparous Lamaze Couples Who Share Delivery and Those Who Do Not." The title of the article "Subjects, data, and videotapes" (Heacock, Souder, & Chastain, 1996), was a clever parallel to the popular film "Sex, lies and videotapes."

The books on style and writing listed in appendix A will prove useful, especially when one is deciding on the format for the report, the general style of writing, and how to cite references.

WRITING FOR PUBLICATION

In addition to preparing a report of your research, you may wish to bring your study to the attention of nurses generally by writing one or more articles based on it for publication in one or more of the professional journals. Before doing so, it would be a good idea for you to look at some recent issues of these journals and note the kind and length of articles they tend to publish; the type of article you write will depend on the journal you select. Some potential authors find it helpful to read several current issues of a journal to get a flavor of what type of material is usually presented.

All professional journals have editorial policies regarding the subject matter of articles they accept for publication. They also have directions or specifications for the preparation of manuscripts that they will send you on request. When you write for these specifications, it is a good idea to inquire whether the editors would be interested in an article on the subject of your study. All journals have space limitations, and if the journal you select has recently carried articles similar to yours, it may not be interested in publishing another one until considerable time has elapsed. In that case, you can query another journal that might be interested. Today, nurse authors have a rather wide range of professional journals from which to choose, including clinical specialty areas, such as *Journal of Obstetric, Gynecologic and Neonatal Nursing* (JOGNN) and *Heart and Lung, The Journal of Critical Care,* the official publication of the American Association of Critical-Care Nurses. Consult the International Nursing Index under "Publications Indexed" for a list of major nursing journals. Swanson, McCloskey, and Bodensteiner (1991) compare 92 journals that provide publishing opportunities for nurses.

If the journal you select expresses interest in your article, follow its style in preparing your manuscript. Many journals now require that an electronic copy of the manuscript be submitted on disk along with the required paper, or hard, copies. Send the editor the number of copies required and always be sure to keep a copy for yourself. Make sure to take all precautions necessary to prevent data loss on your computer. Always make back-up copies.

Many professional journals that report research, *Nursing Research,* for example, have a team of volunteer experts review all manuscripts submitted for publication. In *Scholarly Inquiry for Nursing Practice* they are listed as consulting reviewers. Other journals have manuscripts reviewed by several editors on their regular editorial board or a panel of peer reviewers. Madeline Schmitt (1998), editor of *Research in Nursing and Health,* invites interested peer reviewers to submit letters of intent. She lists the major criteria as (a) evidence of published peer-reviewed, data-based research and (b) a well-written initial manuscript review. Molly Dougherty (1997), editor of *Nursing Research,* discusses factors that go into selecting an editorial review board. Needed are representation within specific dimensions: professional productivity, clinical or other discipline-defining substantive areas, methodologies, analytic approaches, geographical distribution, and expertise to address elements of the journal purpose. According to Dougherty, "The challenge is to select a set of individuals with the expertise mix needed to represent the varied research under way in nursing. The editorial board needs to communicate meaningfully about the direction and content of the journal" (p. 245). It is useful for prospective authors to look at the names, primary institutional affiliation, and expertise of the editorial board of various journals. Most journals list the members of their review board.

In any event, the review takes time, and you may not hear about the disposition of your manuscript for 3 or 4 months. Most journals acknowledge receipt of a manuscript immediately by card or form letter, but the author probably does not hear until much later whether the material has been accepted. Following acceptance, another 6 months or even 1 year may go by before the author sees the article or report in print. Some journals will cite the date when the article was accepted for publication. For example, the length of time from acceptance to publication for articles published in the January/February 1998 issue of *Nursing Research* ranged from 4 to 8 months. Not only does the process of preparing a paper and scheduling it for publication take time, but also some journals always have a number of accepted manuscripts already on hand, and yours must wait its turn. Be patient!

What should you do if your manuscript is declined or if the editors of the journal you have selected suggest that you make major revisions in it? Don't take it as a personal insult. If you can make the suggested revisions, do so, and then resubmit the article. If a journal declines your paper, this does not necessarily mean that you should give up the idea of trying to get it published. As noted earlier, several journals that publish nursing articles are available to you, and rejection by one does not close the door to publication. Select another journal, find out its requirements for articles, look your manuscript over to make sure it meets these requirements, and send it off again. If the journal that rejected your paper gave you the reasons for its rejection, make the suggested changes or corrections before you send it to someone else, if it is possible for you to do so.

It may occur to you to submit your article to more than one journal at a time in order to enlarge your chance of success. This is not considered ethical practice. A great deal of work goes into editorial review and if your article is accepted by one of several journals, the others will be disturbed by your unethical behavior. Also, if you are accepted by more than one journal, what will you do? It is better to select one journal at a time. Of course, submit your manuscript first to the journal that is your first choice, but if you are not their first choice, do not despair. There are enough journals today to try, try again.

Acknowledgments

We would like to add a word here about the good manners of acknowledging others' help. Rarely is your research a solitary, independent activity, whether it be in its funding or in seeking advice and consultation. Many researchers will also acknowledge the assistance of a consulting statistician and their secretary for manuscript preparation. You do not have to make your acknowledgment a laundry list, but it is an appropriate gesture to express gratitude, be it ever so brief and in small type.

Research Presentations

This is a chicken and egg question. Which comes first: presenting your research at a research conference, such as your state's or regional specialty practice nursing society or your own local institution's Sigma Theta Tau research meeting or submitting it for publication? "Getting the kinks out" by presenting your study to peers, whether as a speech or a poster presentation, may provide you with perspectives you had not previously considered. Selby, Tornquist, and Finerty (1988) point out the essentials that will make your research presentation more valuable. "Remember, listeners want to know what you found; that's why they came to hear you instead of waiting to read your study in a journal next year" (Selby et al., 1988, p. 175). Some research conferences may not want to accept research for presentation if it has already been published, so consider that when contemplating what comes first. Although submitting for publication, revision, acceptance, and publication may take the long periods of time we referred to earlier in this chapter, you may want to share your findings for knowledge development, dissemination, and use as soon as possible. Consider presentations at local, state, regional, national, and even international meetings as part of the research process. For example, in the New York University *Center for Continuing Education in Nursing Bulletin* (Spring, 1998) it states that their annual nursing research conference provides a forum for the nursing community to disseminate current knowledge in nursing research. Paper and poster sessions are grouped into common research themes; such as clinical practice, nursing informatics, nursing education, and mental health nursing.

Poster presentations have become increasingly popular at research conferences (Lippman & Ponton, 1989). Rempusheski (1990) has written an excellent "how to" article about the organization, mechanics, and costs of preparing a poster to display findings of QA research or a clinical project. (See appendix A for other good sources.) Presenting a poster provides the researcher with close dialogue with other professional peers, what politicians would call "pressing the flesh." It's a very rewarding way to develop research "pen pals" (even if it is e-mail). Make sure you bring along an adequate supply of your study's abstract and your own professional business cards to distribute.

SUMMARY

Generally, research is not considered complete until it has been disseminated through presentation or publication, thus making results of the study available to others. One of the great needs in nursing today is for nurses generally to read and evaluate reports of research that is being done and to make use of research findings, when indicated, for the improvement of nursing practice. In this chapter we have concentrated on the importance of communicating to the nursing profession, colleagues, and lay public the results of research. Now we are ready to consider the important steps of evaluation and implementation of research findings.

REFERENCES

Barnum, B. (1995). *Writing and getting published: A primer for nurses.* New York: Springer Publishing Co.

Beyerman, K. L. (1987). Developing the motivation to write for publication. *Clinical Nurse Specialist, 1,* 3–6.

Budin, W. (1998). Psychosocial adjustment to breast cancer in unmarried women. *Research in Nursing and Health, 21,* 155–166.

Corbett, J. V. (1987). Making time for writing. *Nursing Outlook, 35,* 198.

Dougherty, M. (1997). Welcome to the editorial board. *Nursing Research, 46,* 245.

Hansell, P., Hughes, C., Caliandro, G., Russo, P., Budin, W., Hartman, B., & Hernandez, O. (1998). The effects of a social support boosting intervention on stress, coping, and social support in caregivers of children with HIV/AIDS. *Nursing Research, 47*(2), 79–86.

Heacock, P., Souder, E., & Chastain, J. (1996). Subjects, data, and videotapes. *Nursing Research, 15,* 336–338.

Hickey, M. (1990). What are the needs of families of critically ill patients? A review of the literature since 1976. *Heart and Lung: The Journal of Critical Care, 19,* 410–415.

Hinshaw, A. S. (1989). Nursing science: The challenge to develop knowledge. *Nursing Science Quarterly, 2,* 162–171.

Hott, J. R. (1980). Best laid plans...pre- and postpartum comparison of self and spouse in primiparous Lamaze couples who share delivery and those who do not. *Nursing Research, 29,* 20–27.

Lippman, D. T., & Ponton, K. S. (1989). Designing a research poster with impact. *Western Journal of Nursing Research, 11,* 477–485.

New York University. (1998, Spring). *Center for Continuing Education in Nursing Bulletin.* New York: Author.

Rempusheski, V. F. (1990). Ask an expert: Resources necessary to prepare a poster for presentation. *Applied Nursing Research, 3,* 134–137.

Schmitt, M. (1998). A new editor [Editorial]. *Research in Nursing and Health, 21*(1), 1.

Selby, M. L., Tornquist, E. M., & Finerty, E. J. (1988). How to present your research. *Nursing Outlook, 37,* 172–175.

Sheridan, D., & Dowdney, D. (1997). *How to write and publish articles in nursing* (2nd ed.). New York: Springer Publishing Co.

Swanson, E. A., McCloskey, J. C., & Bodensteiner, A. (1991). Publishing opportunities for nurses: A comparison of 92 U.S. journals. *Image: Journal of Nursing Scholarship, 23*(1), 33–38.

PART III

Evaluation of Research

12

The Evaluation Process

For nursing research to have the greatest possible impact on nursing and the nursing process, practicing nurses must be familiar with the research that has been carried out and must be able to determine its usefulness. This is one of the most important functions of every nurse. To some it may seem a formidable task, but those who have read the previous chapters of this book already have an introduction to the basic facts about research that are needed to evaluate the studies of others.

The first question one should ask when evaluating a study should be, how much confidence can I place in the findings of the studies reported? One measure of confidence relates to the reputation of the investigator. Is the investigator well known in the field under study? What are the investigator's qualifications for doing the research? Most research reports carry a brief statement about the author or investigator that will enable you to estimate, at least with some degree of confidence, the researcher's qualifications to do the research and the extent to which you can probably rely on these findings. Sometimes a less experienced investigator works under the guidance of a more sophisticated researcher; this should help to substantiate the quality of the work.

Another measure of quality is related to the periodical in which the report is published. Articles submitted to scientific journals are subjected to peer evaluation prior to publication, usually by reviewers or referees who are experts in the subject studied and the research methods used. Although this measure of quality is not foolproof, one can justifiably feel some additional confidence in the reports these journals publish.

In addition to these two measures of quality, nurses must also make their own decisions about the quality and significance of the research reported. To do this you will need a knowledge of the essentials of nursing research, such as are set forth in this text. It will also be helpful to have at least some knowledge of the clinical area involved in the study. Of course, if you are reading it to evaluate the usefulness of the findings in your own practice, you should have a better than average knowledge of the subject under study in the report.

Remember that most research has certain limitations. The purpose of any investigation is to search for truth. All research reflects the state of present knowledge, however, and because of this and because of the limitations in the research process itself, findings rarely include the ultimate answer. The work must be evaluated in terms of how much it enlarges present knowledge and what future investigations it suggests.

A first step in evaluation is careful reading of the report as a whole. A good report will be well-organized around the usual steps in the research procedure, and the information will be logically presented. With minor variations, scientific reports commonly follow the outline suggested in chapter 11. As you read, ask yourself questions about each part of the report.

THE RESEARCH PROBLEM

The first few questions you might ask are, what was the purpose of this study? Why was it done? Does the introduction clearly state the problem investigated? What was the scope of the problem? Is there a theoretical framework? Were the limits of the study clearly indicated? One needs to have a clear understanding of the problem under investigation and the purpose of the research in order to evaluate the soundness of the method used to study it.

Your next question might be, how significant was the problem? This query, of course, relates directly to the purpose of the study. A criticism sometimes heard is that some research has no significance for nursing. For example, the contribution of historical research to clinical practice may be questioned. Brodie (1988), a nurse historian, addresses this in "Voices in Distant Camps: The Gap between Nursing Research and Nursing Practice." Nevertheless, historical research can have significant long-range effects. It can, for example, contribute to better understanding of why nursing took the directions it did at various time periods and how these past actions influenced, and continue to influence, today's decisions regarding the delivery of health care.

It is true, however, that some research may be focused on problems that are more obviously significant than others. How well does the investigator justify the study in this regard? To answer this question and to determine the importance of the study will require that you bring your own judgment to the evaluation process.

THE LITERATURE REVIEW

Once you have determined the problem under study and its significance, an examination of the investigator's review of the literature is in order. How was this review related to the problem studied? Did it lead logically to the hypothesis or the questions raised for study? Sometimes literature reviews have little relevance to the study; the author may report a series of studies in related areas but not tie them in with the present investigation. The literature review should help clarify the problem, identify and relate previous research in the area to this study, and lead logically to the question to be studied. It should also clearly identify the theoretical framework of the research when this is an important aspect of the study. For a "state of the science" in a literature review, read Smeltzer and Whipple (1991). Again, your knowledge of the clinical field involved and of available literature in that field will be helpful in your evaluation of the research. For a concise summary of what a literature review should include, read Haller (1988).

THE HYPOTHESIS

After you have examined the investigator's literature review, you may ask, is the hypothesis or the question to be studied clearly stated? If the research is experimental, are the independent and dependent variables clearly identified? The research question should be one that can be studied with the research tools at hand. Hypotheses such as those stated by Miller and Perry (1990) in their study were clearly appropriate in that the means of collecting the necessary data were available from patient records and self-reports.

Probably at this point you will ask, are all terms specific to the study clearly defined in the report? In many instances, the answer to this question will be very important.

THE RESEARCH METHOD

When you come to the description of the research method used in a report you are evaluating, your questions probably will include, was the method used descriptive, experimental, qualitative, or historical and was it appropriate to the problem studied and the hypothesis made? For example, the hypotheses in the Miller and Perry (1990) study determined the method to be used: a two-group pretest and posttest quasi-experimental design. On the other hand, Schepp's (1991) study, in line with its purpose, was a descriptive survey.

DATA-COLLECTING PROCEDURES

Once the method of collecting data is determined, one evaluates the appropriateness of the procedures used. These should be described in sufficient detail to permit replication of the research. How were the data collected? Was the appropriate tool used? Were the data collected by questionnaire when observation methods should have been used? Was the tool used a well-established one or one devised for the study? Was the validity and reliability of the tool described?

Was the sample appropriate? How was it selected? Was the sample size adequate? Was investigator bias controlled in any way? Were the rights of subjects protected? Did the investigator recognize any flaws or lacks in the procedures used and the possible effects of these deficiencies on the results of the research? Deficiencies do not necessarily negate the study if they are recognized and if the estimation of their effect on the results is calculated by the investigator when presenting the findings. There are few perfect designs, especially in clinical research, in which the complex human situations involved often introduce hard-to-control intervening factors that may have an impact on your best-laid research plans (see Hott, 1980). The purpose in evaluating the design is to determine the extent to which the deficiencies invalidate the findings: They may be so minimal that they have little or no adverse effect on the results of the study.

ANALYSIS OF THE DATA

The data analysis, that is, the presentation of the findings, should be objectively and accurately reported. This may become the most difficult part of the evaluation, especially if sophisticated statistical measures are used. For assistance in making this part of your evaluation, you might reread chapter 8, "Analysis of the Data."

CONCLUSIONS REACHED

In evaluating the conclusions reached by the investigator, consider how far these are justified by the findings. A common error on the part of the beginning investigator is to go beyond the findings of the study in discussing conclusions reached and the general applicability of the study findings. Personal experiences or opinions may be allowed to creep in and contaminate the objectivity of the conclusions. The experienced investigator strives for utmost objectivity, uses restraint in making observations, and expresses necessary reservations in drawing conclusions. Generalizations must not go beyond the evidence presented.

Many reports include a discussion section in which the findings are related to those of other researchers. It is here that implications for nursing, if appropriate, may be made. The investigator's opinion, properly identified, about the significance of the findings for nursing or for further research may be included. Your evaluation of these opinions will be in terms of the appropriateness of the statements concerning the implications. You might ask, did the study expand or extend knowledge? You might also ask, can I use the findings of this study in my own work? If so, how?

Several additional sources, "Cognitive Skills and Development Competencies for Conducting Research Critiques" (Millor et al., 1991), "The Research Critique" (Beck, 1990), and "Demystifying Research: A Guide for the Perinatal Educator" (Budin, 1996), are highly recommended to help consumers of research with the critique process. For another valuable example of how the quality of research was measured using Duffy's (1985) RAC, you are urged to review Brown's (1990) "Quality of Reporting in Diabetes Patient Education Research: 1954–1986."

SUMMARY

Although not all nurses will become involved in research as investigators or as research assistants, all do have a responsibility for making appropriate use of the findings of research in their work. This chapter has briefly outlined some of the factors in evaluating the quality of research and in estimating the value of research findings for the improvement of nursing care, a major objective of nursing research.

REFERENCES

Beck, C. T. (1990). The research critique. *Journal of Obstetric, Gynecologic and Neonatal Nursing, 19,* 18–22.

Brodie, B. (1988). Voices in distant camps: The gap between nursing research and nursing practice. *Journal of Professional Nursing, 4,* 320–328.

Brown, S. A. (1990). Quality of reporting in diabetes patient education research: 1954–1986. *Research in Nursing and Health, 13,* 53–62.

Budin, W. (1996). Demystifying research: A guide for the perinatal educator. *Journal of Perinatal Education, 5*(3), 59–62.

Duffy, M. E. (1985). A research appraisal checklist for evaluating nursing research reports. *Nursing and Health Care, 6,* 539–547.

Haller, K. B. (1988). Conducting a literature review. *Maternal Child Nursing, 13,* 148.

Hott, J. R. (1980). Best laid plans . . . Pre- and postpartum comparison of self and spouse in primiparous Lamaze couples who share delivery and those who do not. *Nursing Research, 29,* 20–27.
Miller, K. M., & Perry, P. A. (1990). Relaxation technique and postoperative pain in patients undergoing cardiac surgery. *Heart and Lung: Journal of Critical Care, 19,* 136–146.
Millor, G. K., Levin, R. F., Carter, E., Doswell, W., Jacobson, L., & Shortridge, L. M. (1991). Cognitive skills and development competencies for conducting research critiques. *Journal of the New York State Nurses Association, 22,* 12–16.
Schepp, K. G. (1991). Factors influencing the coping efforts of mothers of hospitalized children. *Nursing Research, 40,* 42–46.
Smeltzer, S. C., & Whipple, B. (1991). Women and HIV infection. *Image: Journal of Nursing Scholarship, 23,* 249–256.

Appendix A

Useful Reference Sources on Writing and Presenting Research

American Psychological Association (1994). *Publication manual of the American Psychological Association* (4th ed.). Washington, DC: Author.

Barnum, B. (1995). *Writing and getting published: A primer for nurses.* New York: Springer Publishing Co.

Beyerman, K. L. (1987). Developing the motivation to write for publication. *Clinical Nurse Specialist, 1,* 3–6.

Brooks-Brunn, J. (1996). Poster etiquette. *Applied Nursing Research, 9,* 97–99.

Carpinello, S., & Caley, L. (1993). Preparing research results for journal submissions. *Journal of New York State Nurses Association, 24*(1), 5–7.

Chicago Manual of Style (14th ed.) (1993). Chicago: University of Chicago Press.

Chinn, P. L. (1992). From the editor: Challenging, visionary, innovative. *Nursing Outlook, 40*(4), 148–149.

Day, R. A. (1983). *How to write and publish a scientific paper* (2nd ed.). Philadelphia: ISI.

Fitzpatrick, J. (1995). The making of a manuscript [editorial]. *Applied Nursing Research, 8,* 1–2.

Fitzpatrick, J. (1998). *Encyclopedia of nursing research.* New York: Springer Publishing Co.

Fondiller, S. (1992). *The writer's workbook.* New York: National League for Nursing.

Jackle, M. (1989). Presenting research to nurses in clinical practice. *Applied Nursing Research, 2,* 191–193.

Lippman, D., & Ponton, K. (1998). Designing a research poster with impact. *Western Journal of Nursing Research, 11,* 477–485.

Locke, L. (1987). *Proposals that work: A guide for planning dissertations and grant proposals.* Newbury Park, CA: Sage.

Maggio, R. E. (1987). *Nonsexist word finder: A dictionary of gender free usage.* Phoenix, AZ: Oryx Press.

Martin, P. (1994). Poster session tips for the novice viewer. *Applied Nursing Research, 7,* 208–210.

Miracle, V., & King, K. (1994). Presenting research: Effective paper presentations and impressive poster presentations. *Applied Nursing Research, 7,* 147–151.

Rempusheski, V. (1990). Resources necessary to prepare a poster for presentation. *Applied Nursing Research, 3,* 134–137.
Robinson, A., & Notter, L. (1982). *Clinical writing for health professionals.* Bowie, MD: Robert J. Brady.
Ryan, N. M. (1989). Developing and presenting a research poster. *Applied Nursing Research, 2,* 52–55.
Selby, M. L., Tornquist, E. M., & Finerty, E. J. (1988). How to present your research. *Nursing Outlook, 37,* 172–175.
Sherbinski, L., & Stroup, D. (1992) Developing a poster for disseminating research findings. *Journal of the American Association of Nurse Anesthetists, 60,* 567–572.
Sheridan, D., & Dowdney, D. (1997). *How to write and publish articles in nursing* (2nd ed.). New York: Springer Publishing Co.
Sigma Theta Tau International. (1984). *Why write? Why publish? A collection of papers from the Sigma Theta Tau writers' seminars.* Indianapolis, IN: Author.
Skillin, M. & Gay, R. (1986). *Words into type* (3rd ed.). Englewood Cliffs, NJ: Prentice-Hall.
Swanson, E. A., McCloskey, J. C., & Bodensteiner, A. (1991). Publishing opportunities for nurses: A comparison of 92 U.S. journals. *Image: Journal of Nursing Scholarship, 23*(1), 33–38.
Tornquist, E. M. (1986). *From proposal to publication: An informal guide to writing about nursing research.* Menlo Park, CA: Addison Wesley.
Turabian, K. (1987). *Manual for writers of term papers, theses, and dissertations* (5th ed.). Chicago: University of Chicago Press.
Ventura, M. (1992). Guidelines for writing for publication. *Journal of the New York State Nurses Association, 23*(2).
Williams, J. (1990). *Style: Toward clarity and grace.* Chicago: University of Chicago Press.
Zinsser, W. (1990). *On writing well* (4th ed.). New York: Harper & Row.

AND DON'T FORGET THESE "OLDIES BUT GOODIES"

Bernstein, T. (1997). *Dos, don'ts & maybes of English usage.* New York: Times Books.
Strunk, W., & White, E. (1979). *The elements of style* (3rd ed.). New York: Macmillan.

Appendix B

Useful References for Finding Funds for Nursing Research

Bauer, D., & American Association of Colleges of Nursing. (1988). *The complete grants source book for nursing and health.* B. K. Redman, Ed., R. Lmothe; Managing Ed.). New York: American Council on Education & Macmilian.

Kelley, J. A., & Gray, J. T. (1990). Elements of grantsmanship: The process; the art. *Nursing and Health Care, 11,* 246–352.

Kemp, C. (1991). A practical approach to writing successful grant proposals. *Nurse Practitioner, 16,* 51, 55–56.

National Institute for Nursing Research. (1995). *Facts About Funding.* NINR, National Institutes of Health, Building 31, Room 5B03, Bethesda, MD, 20892. Contains good bibliography of helpful articles and covers the types of research and research awards available through NINR and NIH.

Nursing Diagnosis Newsletter. (1989, Winter). Nursing research at NIH: How a nursing research grant is made. pp. 4–7.

Redman, B. K. (1988). *The complete grants source book for nursing and health.* New York: Macmilian.

Scholarships and Loans for Nursing Education. National League for Nursing, 340 Hudson Street, New York, New York, 10014 ($12.95). Call 1-800-669-1656, ext. 138. Includes fellowships, traineeships, and grants for research and postdoctoral studies.

Toliver, J. C., & Toliver, A. P. (1988). Nursing research: How to prepare a competitive research grant application. *Journal of the National Black Nurses' Association, 2*(2), 26–35.

Tornquist, E., & Funk, S. (1990). How to write a research grant proposal. *Image: Journal of Nursing Scholarship, 22*(1), 44–51.

ADDITIONAL SOURCES

1. Check with national and local Sigma Theta Tau chapter.
2. Check with national and local American Heart Association and American Diabetes Association.

3. Check with your institution for intramural grants that they might fund.
4. Contact your alumnae associations for possible funding.
5. Check with pharmaceutical companies to see what kinds of projects they fund.
6. Check with The Foundation Center, located at 888 Seventh Avenue, New York, New York 10106 for grants. Computer databases can be accessed through the Foundation Center (phone DIALOG - 415-858-2700 or phone The Foundation Center). Also, The Foundation Center publishes a number of excellent directories. Examples are:

   AIDS funding: A guide to giving by foundations and charitable organizations. December 1998/ISBN 0-87954-7235/$75.00.

   Foundation fundamentals: A guide for grantseekers (5th ed.). Edited by Mitchell F. Nauffts & Judith B. Margolin (Eds.). December 1994/ISBN 0-87954-5437/$24.95.

   National guide to funding for children, youth, and families. April 1997/ ISBN 0-87954-7111/$150.00. Published biennially.

   New York state foundations: A comprehensive directory (4th ed.). May 1995/ISBN 0-87954-6093/$175.00. Published biennially.

   The Foundation directory. Part 2. A guide to grant programs $25,000 to $100,000 (20th ed.). March 1998/ISBN 0-87954-7626/$185.00. Published biennially.

   The national guide to funding in aging (4th ed.). November 1994/ISBN 0-87954-5593/$80.

   The national guide to funding in health (3rd ed.). March 1993/ISBN 0-87954-379-5.

GRANTS FUNDING SOURCES

Name	Address
National Institute for Nursing Research	NIH/Public Health Service Rm. B2E17, Bldg. 38A Bethesda, MD 20894
Adolescent Family Life Research Grants	Office of Adolescent Pregnancy Programs—DHHS HHH Building, Rm. 736E 200 Independence Ave., SW Washington, DC 20201
Occupational Safety and Health Research Grants	National Institute for Occupational Safety and Health 1600 Clifton Road, NE Atlanta, GA 30333

Alcohol Research Programs	Div. Extramural Research, NIAAA Public Health Service, DHHS 5600 Fishers Lane Rockville, MD 20857
Drug Abuse Research Programs	National Institute on Drug Abuse 5600 Fishers Lane Room 11A-3 Rockville, MD 20857
Minority Biomedical Research Support	Division of Research Resources National Institutes of Health Bethesda, MD 20892
Academic Research Enhancement Award	Office of Special Programs and Initiatives Office of Extramural Research Training National Institutes of Health Bethesda, MD 20892
Health Financing Research, Demonstrations, and Experiments	Office of Research and Development HCFA—DHHS 6325 Security Blvd. Baltimore, MD 21207
Research for Mothers and Children	Office of Grants & Contracts National Institute of Child Health & Human Development National Institutes of Health Bethesda, MD 20892
Aging Research	National Institute on Aging National Institutes of Health Bethesda, MD 20892
National Institute of Handicapped Research	Department of Education Mail Stop 2304 400 Maryland Ave., SW Washington, DC 20202

Private

Name	**Address**
American Nurses Foundation	American Nurses Association 600 Maryland Ave., Suite 100 Washington, DC 20024

Sigma Theta Tau International Grants Program	Sigma Theta Tau International 550 West North Street Indianapolis, IN 46202
AARP	AARP Andrus Foundation 601 E. Street, NW Washington, DC 20049
March of Dimes	Grants Administration 1275 Mamaroneck Avenue White Plains, NY 10605
American Cancer Society	Research Grants Mary LeMahieu, Grants Administrator Research Department 1599 Clifton Road, NE Atlanta, GA 30329
Diabetes Research & Education Foundation, Inc.	Executive Director P.O. Box 6168 Bridgewater, NJ 08807-9998

Note: Check Web sites included in appendix E for additional information on funding agencies.

Appendix C

Writing a Research Abstract

GENERAL GUIDELINES

An abstract is a brief summarization of a research project that emphasizes four general categories of information: what was done, how it was done, the results obtained, and how the author interprets them. Authors must address each and every one of these categories in order for an abstract to be considered complete. Subtopics need to be addressed within these four general categories, as well. If a list of subtopics is provided in a call for abstracts then the prudent author discusses each one in the order suggested, which usually reflects the sequence of the research process.

If completeness is the first challenge of abstract writers, then brevity is the second. Abstracts often need to be composed with stringent and inviolate work limitations. A 200–250 word limit is common. Sometimes authors are provided with a form on which the abstract is required to fit. If no word or space limitations are required, authors should still aim for brevity. Additionally, the final product must be grammatically and typographically correct, free of jargon and colloquialisms. Acronyms should be defined and used sparingly, but never in the title. Use a high quality printer and take care that the abstract makes a good visual impression.

Abstract writing is highly stylized. The combination of thoroughness and brevity is a challenging one, especially when it comes to a project in which the author is thoroughly invested and knowledgeable. Remember that all the other researchers submitting abstracts are undergoing the same difficult mental process: reducing work that may have taken years to complete to a few pithy paragraphs.

(Reprinted with permission from the New York State Nurses Association Council on Nursing Research)

SPECIFIC NYSNA GUIDELINES

Please include information about all of the following items in your abstract:

Title: The goal should be a specific, concise, and interesting title that clearly indicates the nature of the research. The title must convey the topic but may also reveal the design used and the subjects.

Purpose of the research: This section should establish the importance of the problem addressed, the rationale for the study and exactly what the author intended to accomplish. Attempt to make a logical connection between the purposes and earlier work in this area, and the conceptual/theoretical framework used in the study (if any).

Hypothesis(es) or research questions: Hypotheses are formal predictions about how the variables studied will be related. They should logically flow from what is already known about the topic. Space will not allow for hypotheses to be listed verbatim; their general thrust must be summarized. Sometimes not enough information exists to permit hypothesis construction. In addition, qualitative studies are by nature hypothesis generating rather than testing. In both cases the author should summarize the research questions answered by the research or the hypotheses generated for future testing.

Significance for nursing: Indicate how the research will improve nursing practice specifically and/or advance the profession as a whole.

Research design: This section should reveal the overall organizational plan for the study. The specific type of quantitative or qualitative methods should be identified.

Population or sample: Most research entails samples rather than populations. Make it clear which is being used in the study. Reveal the characteristics of subjects (persons, groups, organizations), their number, the recruitment strategy, and the study setting.

Data-collection methods: Describe who collected the data, and the type of tools or research interventions used. Validity and/or reliability information may be important depending on the nature of the study.

Methods of analysis: Discuss the data analysis methods used. Levels of statistical significance should be defined and indicated by conventional symbols if conducting a quantitative study.

Research findings: This section describes what was revealed and not revealed as a result of the study. Present the factual outcomes of the study.

Implications of the findings for nursing: Tie the other sections of the paper together and give them meaning in this part of the abstract. Discuss the results in light of previous work, the study's conceptual framework, and methods used. Limitations of the study may be mentioned. Conclusions are frequently stated in tentative terms. Relate the findings to nursing practice or education or the profession as a whole. Make specific recommendations when appropriate.

REFERENCES

Burns, N., & Grove, S. K. (1993). *The practice of nursing research: Conduct, critique and utilization* (2nd ed.). Philadelphia: W. B. Saunders.

LoBiondo-Wood, G., & Haber, J. (Eds.). (1993). *Nursing research: Methods, critical appraisal and utilization.* St. Louis: Mosby Yearbook.

Pruitt, B. A., & Mason, A. D. (1991) Writing an effective abstract. In H. Troidl (Ed.). *Principles & practice of research: Strategies for surgical investigators* (2nd ed.). (pp. 380–383). New York: Springer-Verlag.

Woods, N. F., & Catanzaro, M. (1988). *Nursing research: Theory and practice.* Toronto: C. V. Mosby.

Appendix D

Overview of Research Serials in Nursing

Title	Publisher	Focus
Annual Review of Nursing Research	Springer Publishing Co. 536 Broadway New York, NY 10012	Yearly updates on research in four broad subject areas; practice, education, care delivery systems, and the profession
Applied Nursing Research	W. B. Saunders Curtis Center Independence Square West Philadelphia, PA 19106	Clinical implication of nursing research
Canadian Journal of Nursing Research	School of Nursing McGill University 3506 University St. Montreal, QC H3A 2A7	Broad subject base; detailed original research; abstracts in English and French; no geographic limitation on submitters
Communicating Nursing Research	Western Institute of Nursing PO Drawer P Boulder, CO 80301	Annual proceedings of the Western Society for Research in Nursing Conference
International Journal of Nursing Studies	Pergamon Press, Inc. Maxwell House Fairview Park Elmsford, NY 10523	Primarily in issues related topics of nursing research
Journal of Nursing Measurement	Springer Publishing Co. 536 Broadway New York, NJ 10012	Contains information on research tools/ instrumentation

Reprinted with permission from the New York State Nurses Association Council on Nursing Research.

Nursing Research	American Journal of Nursing Co. 555 W. 57th St. New York, NY 10019	Broad subject base; detailed original research
Nursing Science Quarterly	Chestnut House Publishing PO Box 22492 Philadelphia, PA 15222	Broad subject base; integration of theory, research and practice provides a balance between concrete and abstract
Rehabilitation Nursing Research	Association of Rehabilitation Nurses 4700 W. Lake Ave. Glenview, Il 60025	Specific subject with detailed original research; also contains resource views, grant information
Research in Nursing Health	John Wiley & Sons 605 Third Ave. New York, NY 10158	Broad subject base; detailed original research with a focus on clinical implications
Scholarly Inquiry for Nursing Practice	Springer Publishing Co. 536 Broadway New York, NY 10012	Broad subject base; deals with the integration of theory, research, and practice
Western Journal of Nursing Research	Sage Publications 2111 W. Hillcrest Dr. Newbury Park, CA 91320	Broad subject base; detailed original research; in addition contains abstracts/news about ongoing/completed research

The following selected clinical nursing journals are noted for their inclusion of research articles. The materials generally contain more than 50% research articles.

Journal	**Publisher**
American Journal of Critical Care	American Association of Critical-Care Nurses 101 Columbia Aliso Viejo, CA 92656
Cancer Nursing	Raven Press, Ltd. 1185 Avenue of the Americas New York, NY 10036
Cardiovascular Nursing	American Heart Association, Inc. 7272 Greenville Avenue Dallas, TX 75231-4596
Computers in Nursing	J. B. Lippincott Co. 100 Insurance Way Suite 114 Hagerstown, MD 21740

Diabetes Educator	American Association of Diabetes Educators 444 N. Michigan Avenue Suite 1240 Chicago, IL 60611-3901
Heart & Lung: Journal of Critical Care	Mosby-Year Book, Inc. 11830 Westline Industrial Drive St. Louis, MO 63146-3318
Image: Journal of Nursing Scholarship	Sigma Theta Tau International Image Publication Office Honor Society of Nursing, Inc. Indianapolis, IN 46202
Issues in Mental Health Nursing	Taylor & Francis 1900 Frost Road Suite 101 Bristol, PA 19007
Journal of Advanced Nursing	Blackwell Scientific Publications, Ltd. PO Box 87 Oxford OX2 ODT, England
Journal of Continuing Education	SLACK, Inc. 6900 Grove Road Thorofare, NJ 08086
Journal of Nurse-Midwifery	American College of Nurse Midwives 1522 K Street Washington, DC 20005
Journal of Nursing Education	SLACK, Inc. 6900 Grove Road Thorofare, NJ
Journal of Pediatric Nursing: Nursing Care of Children and Families	W. B. Saunders Co. The Curtis Center Independence Square West Philadelphia, PA 19106-3399
Journal of Transcultural Nursing	Transcultural Nursing Society 36600 Schoolcraft Road Livonia, MI 48150
Maternal–Child Nursing Journal	Nursecom, Inc. 1211 Locust Street Philadelphia, PA 19107
Nurse Anesthesia	Appleton & Lange 25 Van Zant Street East Norwalk, CT 06855
Oncology Nursing Forum	Oncology Nursing Press, Inc. 501 Holiday Drive Pittsburgh, PA 15220-2749

Public Health Nursing	Blackwell Scientific Publications, Ltd. 238 Main Street Suite 501 Cambridge, MA 02142
Qualitative Health Research	Sage Publication, Inc. 2455 Teller Road Thousand Oaks, CA 91320
Rehabilitation Nursing	*Association of Rehabilitation Nurses* 5700 Old Orchard Road 1st Floor Skokie, IL 60077-1057

Appendix E

Selected Internet Web Sites for Nursing-Research-Related Activities

(Note: These addresses are subject to change)

Agency for Health Care Policy and Research (AHCPR)
http://www.ahcpr.gov
Evidence-based health care information

Alan Guttmacher Institute
http://www.agi-usa.org
Many publications and periodicals available, online information about reproductive health research

American Academy of Nurse Practitioners (AANP)
http://www.aanp.org
Information available on the AANP

American Association of Colleges of Nursing (AACN)
http://www.aacn.nche.edu
A variety of information on standards and position statements

American Association of Critical-Care Nurses
http://www.aacn.org

American Association for the History of Nursing (AAHN)
http://www.members.aol.wom/nsghistory/index.html

American Association of Legal Nurse Consultants
http://www.aalnc.org/index.htm

American College of Nurse Practitioners
http://www. Nurse.org/acnp

American Holistic Nurses Association
http://www.ahna.org

American Journal of Nursing Company Online
http://www.ajn.org:80
Index and table of contents for numerous journals

American Nurses Association
http://www.nursing.world.org
ANA Homepage. Links to State Nurses Associations.

American Psychiatric Nurses Association
http://www.apna.org
Information useful to psychiatric nurses

Association of Reproductive Health Professions
http://www.arhp.org

Association for Womens Health, Obstetric, and Neonatal Nurses (AWHONN)
http://www.awhonn.org

Best Practice Network
http://www.best4health.org
Research-based clinical innovations

CancerNet-International Cancer Information Center
http://cancernet.nci.nih.gov
Information for health professionals, the general public, and Cancer researchers

Centers for Disease Control and Prevention
http://www.cdc.gov
All material published by the CDC, including guidelines

Community of Science
http://www.cos.com
Database providing funding information from federal and state governments, foundations, professional societies, associations, corporations, and other scientific organizations

Cumulative Index for Nursing and Allied Health Literature (CINAHL)
http://www.cinahl.com
Database for searching nursing and allied health journals

Department of Health and Human Services
http://www.os.dhhs.gov

HospitalWeb
http://neuro-www.mgh.harvard.edu/hospitalweb.hclk

Kinsey Institute
http://www.indiana.edu/~kinsey
For research in sex, gender, and reproduction

National Center for Health Statistics
http://www.cdc.gov/nchswww/index.htm
Provides access to a variety of sites for health statistics

National Institute for Nursing Research (NINR)
http://www.hih.gov/ninr/index.html
Information about research solicited and funded by the NINR

National Institutes of Health (NIH)
http://www.nih.gov

National League for Nursing (NLN)
http://www.nln.org
Information on membership, councils, and accreditation

National Library of Medicine's MEDLINE
http://www.nlm.hih.gov/databases/freemedl.html
Provides access for a free MEDLINE search

Nursing Net
http://www.nursingnet.org
Offers links to nursing-related journals and professional organizations as well as a forum for exchange of ideas

Nursing World
http://www.nursingworld.org
The official site of the American Nurses Association; offers information about the organization's activities, links to state nurses associations

OncoLink
http://cancer.med.upenn.edu
A comprehensive cancer site directed toward health care providers, patients, and their supporters

QualPage
http://www.oise.on.ca/~jnorris/welcom.html
Judy Norris'Home Page: resource of qualitative research

Robert Wood Johnson Foundation
www.rwjf.org
Information on grants and programs

Sigma Theta Tau International
www.stti.iupui.edu
Home page with links to Virginia Henderson Library, Registry of Nurse Researchers, and Online Journal of Nursing Scholarship; also has information about conferences, grants, and other activities

US Department of Health and Human Services
www.os.dhhs.gov
Information about biomedical research, health services research, and health statistics

Virginia Henderson International Nursing Library
www.stti.iupui.edu/library/
Databases for registries of nurse researchers and research projects

Sample Listserves (For a comprehensive list see Nicoll, 1998, p. 196)

NURSERES:
Provides a discussion list on nursing research and related health and professional issues
To subscribe, please send an e-mail to: listserv@kentvm.kent.edu
In the body of your message please type: subscribe NURSERES First name Last name

Martha Rogers Online
Provides discussion on the Science of Unitary Human Beings
Martha E. Rogers listserve is called merogers-center.
To subscribe, please send an e-mail to: listproc@lists.nyu.edu
In the body of your message please type: subscribe merogers-center First name Last name.

Women's Health Chat
Menopause Discussion Group
To subscribe, please send an e-mail to: Menopaus@PSUHMC.bitnet
In the body of your message please type: Subscribe menop. First name Last name

Glossary of Selected Terms*

abstract—a short (less than 200 words long), one-page summary of a research proposal or article.

alpha level—level of significance; often set at 0.05, 0.01, or 0.001.

analysis of variance (ANOVA)—a statistical test used to compare the means of two or more groups by comparing the variance between groups with the variance within groups.

applied research—seeks to find solutions to practical problems; for example, clinical research on problems in nursing practice. *See* research.

assumptions—facts generally accepted as true or correct.

basic research—research that seeks to advance scientific knowledge by establishing new knowledge or facts and developing fundamental theories or principles. The findings of basic research may not be immediately applicable in the solution of problems but may lead to further research. Also called pure research. *See* research.

case study—an in-depth study involving only one subject; occasionally used in qualitative nursing research.

chi-square (χ^2)—a statistical test of significance of data obtained. It is the sum of the quotients obtained by dividing the square of the differences between the observed and theoretical or expected frequencies by the theoretical frequencies.

---

* The *Encyclopedia of Nursing Research* (1998) by Fitzpatrick and published by Springer Publishing Co. presents key terms and concepts in nursing research comprehensively explained by 200 expert contributors. It can be referred to for more detail about terms listed in this glossary.

conceptual definition—provides the reader with a clear description of the meaning of the variable. It is similar to a dictionary definition.

confounding variables—uncontrolled variables that can interfere with the findings of a study. See extraneous variables.

content analysis categories—appropriate subject headings or classifications that an investigator establishes for the purpose of organizing data collected in a study.

content validity—validity of a data-collecting instrument that is established by pointing out the authority for the items used in a questionnaire or checklist.

control variable—a factor in a study that is held constant so as not to intervene and influence the results; for example, age or income of the subjects or type of surgery performed on them. *See* variable.

convenience sample—choosing the most easily and readily accessible people (or places) to be subjects (or units) in a study.

correlation—a measure of degree of relationship between the variables studied. The computed values fall between a +1 and −1. The closer to +1 or −1 they fall, the higher will be the degree of relationship or correlation of the variables.

correlational survey—a survey used to collect data from a group on two or more variables to estimate the relationship between the variables.

criterion measure—a characteristic quality or attribute used to measure the effect of an independent variable on the subjects under study.

criterion variable—*see* dependent variable.

critical incident technique—a method of obtaining data from study subjects' written reports of previous experiences or incidents in their lives that are related to the matter under study.

cross-sectional survey—a survey used to collect comparative data on two or more groups at the same point in time but at different points in the experience of the groups.

data—facts or phenomena. In research, the term commonly refers to the facts observed or obtained in some systematic way (the singular of data is datum).

deductive reasoning—the development of logical answers or conclusions from reliable premises. It starts with general propositions and uses these to derive conclusions; that is, it goes from the general to the particular.

Delphi technique—a special kind of survey using a panel of experts to obtain a consensus on a special topic. Opinions are solicited by mail rather than by the usual group discussion method. It has the advantage of fostering expression of independent opinion.

dependent variable—the variable under observation by the investigator, who wishes to note the effect on it of the introduction of an independent variable. Sometimes called the criterion variable.

descriptive research—present-oriented research that seeks to accurately describe what is and to analyze the facts obtained in relation to the problem under study. It may lead to theories or hypotheses to be tested experimentally.

documentary research—*see* historical research.

empirical—name given to a method of testing or verifying a hypothesis by means of observation or experience. In empirical research, the observations are systematically controlled.

ethnography—a qualitative approach to research in which the investigator learns about a particular culture or situation by becoming a part of the culture or situation under investigation.

experimental research—future-oriented research that tests a hypothesis or hypotheses by setting up a controlled situation and then manipulating it to determine the effect of the manipulation. The design for experimental research consists of control groups and experimental groups that are tested before and after the manipulation of the experimental group or groups. Also called explanatory research.

exploratory study—a preliminary study designed to help refine the problem, develop or refine hypotheses, or test and refine the data-collecting methods. Also called pilot study.

external criticism—investigation to determine whether data collected for a historical study are what they purport to be (authorship, date, etc.).

extraneous variables—variables that can affect the measurement of the study variables or relationships among variables. *See* confounding variables.

face validity—validity of a data-collecting instrument that is assumed after simple inspection of the items on a questionnaire or checklist.

field work—notes or diaries recording an investigator's special area of interest and observations; used by anthropologists to study cultures or groups of people; conducted "in the field," noting subjects in their usual roles.

forced-choice arrangement—*see* Q-sort technique.

frequencies or frequency distribution—a way of ordering data to show the number of subjects for each value or score in a study.

grounded theory—a method in which data collection and analysis are concurrent and ongoing, collecting more specific data based on analysis of the initial data.

Hawthorne effect—when participants in a research study change their behavior not because of a treatment but because they know they are participating in a study.

hermeneutics—a philosophy of science and a method of interpretation of meaning. A phenomenological approach that emphasizes understanding the meaning of experience from the individual's perspective.

historical research—past-oriented research that seeks facts that will help one to interpret and understand past events and their influences. The method used is systematic documentation of the evidence and evaluation of its authenticity.

hypothesis—a statement of predicted relationships between the factors, or variables, under study. It is the tentative deduction usually made as a first step in research (the plural of hypothesis is hypotheses).

independent variable—the variable the investigator manipulates or introduces into the situation. Sometimes called the manipulated variable.

inductive reasoning—the development of logical answers or generalizations by explaining relationships based on facts obtained through observation. Starts with particular situations and goes to general propositions.

inferential statistics—statistics commonly used to test hypotheses by making inferences from a sample to a population.

institutional review board (IRB)—of hospital or school whose primary responsibility is to review all research involving human subjects.

internal criticism—investigation to determine the accuracy of statements in authenticated data that have been collected for a historical study.

interrater reliability—the degree of agreement or consistency between two raters who are independently rating a behavior.

interval data—data representing points on a scale (e.g., body temperature readings).

interview—verbal questioning to collect data.

level of significance—refers to the probability that differences between sets of data are due to chance.

Likert scale—items that usually ask participants if they strongly agree, agree, are neutral, disagree, or strongly disagree with a statement. These items are assumed to yield interval data.

logic—a method of reasoning; a science involved in the development of principles governing inference.

longitudinal survey—a survey that collects data over a period of time for use in studying changes that occur as a result of the experiences occurring or introduced during a specified time period. Also called prospective study.

manipulated variable—*see* independent variable.

mean—the score obtained by adding all the scores or values and dividing this sum by the total number of scores or values; a measure of central tendency.

median—the exact middle score or value in a distribution of scores, obtained by separating the scores or values into an upper and lower half; a measure of central tendency.

meta-analysis—a technique that summarizes and synthesizes multiple variables in similar small studies in research data.

mode—the score or value that occurs most frequently in a distribution of scores or values; a measure of central tendency.

nominal data—data that consist of names or categories of discrete things or conditions (sex, race, diagnosis).

normal curve—a bell-shaped curve showing how values or scores cluster. In a normal distribution, approximately 68% of all scores will fall between a +1 and a –1 standard deviation; approximately 95% will fall between +2 and –2 standard deviations; almost all will fall between +3 and –3 standard deviations.

null hypothesis—a hypothesis that predicts that there will be no significant differences between the results of measures testing control and experimental groups following manipulation of the experimental group. It is related to the statistical test to be used. Rejection of the null hypothesis indicates that there is a statistically significant difference (or differences) between the groups examined.

observation—a method of collecting data by means of one or more persons who observe and record the activity or behavior being studied.

operational definition—provides a clear description of how a variable is observed or measured.

opinionnaire—*see* questionnaire.

ordinal data—data ranked on a qualitative scale on the basis of some specific criterion, that is, arranged in relative order (for example, higher or lower, more or less) on the criterion.

participant-observer—relates to role of investigator in anthropological studies, wherein the investigator becomes a part of the situation under study.

phenomenological approach—a method designed to understand the world of the subjects as they themselves see it. It is appropriate for gaining insight into an area where there is not much existing research and points up areas that may lend themselves to further examination; a form of qualitative research in that it is descriptive and inductive in nature.

phenomenology—the study of human experience that focuses on the process of understanding human behavior and experience.

pilot study—*see* exploratory study.

primary source—a data source that provides direct evidence of an actual event. May be published or unpublished. Examples: the letters of the individual whose life is being studied; an actual tape recording of a meeting.

proposition—a term used in logic to indicate a statement that characterizes something as true or false. A statement of a relationship.

prospective study—*see* longitudinal survey.

Q-sort technique—a method of obtaining data about attitudes; a forced-choice method of rating. Subjects sort cards into a specified number of piles according to the rating the subject has given the object or behavior listed on the card. The number of cards that can be placed in each pile creates an arrangement similar to the normal curve.

qualitative research method—organization and interpretation of observations that provide a more holistic view of the subject's experiences without limiting questions or responses. Relies less on numbers and measurements and more on nursing strategies, interpersonal communication techniques, intuition, and collaboration between nurse and patient/client to discover underlying relationships.

quantitative analysis—using numerical data through statistical procedures to describe and assess relationships between and among them.

quasi-experimental—a study in which Ss cannot be randomly assigned and in which a control group may be missing; not a true experiment.

questionnaire—a paper and pencil method of gathering data from subjects in a study. Data sought usually involve the knowledge, attitudes, observations, or experiences of the subjects. When opinions are sought, the instrument used may be called an opinionnaire.

random sample—a sample in which everyone in the group to be sampled has an equal chance or probability of being selected.

range—the distance between the top and the bottom scores or values in a distribution of scores or values.

rating scale—a method of obtaining a numerical or verbal rating of data that measures such value judgments as attitudes, satisfactions, or other types of subjective response.

ratio level data—highest level of measurement. Ratio data have same properties as interval data however the value of zero means the total absence of a quality.

reliability—refers to the stability and repeatability of the data collection instrument. Reliable instruments obtain consistent results when reused.

research—a systematic inquiry to discover facts or test theories in order to obtain valid answers to questions raised or solutions for problems identified.

sample—a selection of individuals from the total population of a particular class of individuals (e.g., the selection of a group of registered nurses in one state in the United States from the total population of registered nurses in that state).

scientific method—a systematic method employed in study or research in which a problem is identified; a hypothesis (or hypotheses) is made; and data are gathered, systematically arranged, and interpreted in order to test the hypothesis empirically.

secondary source—a data source that is one or more steps removed from the actual event described. A history of an event may contain material from primary sources, but it is itself a secondary source.

serendipity—accidental discovery of valuable findings while the investigator is carrying out a study related to something else.

Standard Deviation—a measure of the variability of scores or values about the mean. See normal curve.

standard error—an estimate of sampling error using a statistical formula. It is an estimate of the normal distribution of all the means that would be obtained if the study were replicated using all samples in the population under study. The standard error of the mean is obtained by dividing the standard deviation of the mean of the sample by the square root of the number in the sample.

statistical inference—a method of statistical analysis used to make inferences about data that is, to determine whether differences between sets of data are significant and to make generalizations that apply to larger populations.

stratified random sample—a sample that has been randomized according to some added factor(s) (e.g., age, religious affiliation). *See* sample, random sample.

structured interview—an interview that follows a set pattern of questioning; used for obtaining more objective data than can be obtained with open-ended questions.

symbols—frequently used in research; some commonly used are

r	correlation	$>$	greater than	α	alpha
p	probability	χ^2	chi-square	F	F-ratio used in ANOVA
$<$	less than	Σ	sum	R^2	multiple regression

tests of significance—statistical methods of determining whether an observed difference in two sets of data is small and therefore not significant, or large and therefore significant.

theoretical framework—provides the theoretical approach to an investigation. The hypothesis and design of the research will be related to the theory selected.

theory—an explanation of facts, or a set of propositions, used as principles to explain a particular class of phenomena.

***t*-test**—a statistical test of significance to determine differences between means of small, randomly selected samples. *t* is equal to the difference between sample and population means divided by the standard error of the difference in sample means.

triangulation—combines both quantitative and qualitative research such as different perspectives in data analysis, multiple sources of data, multiple observers, and two or more methods of data collection.

unstructured interview—an interview that uses open-end questions to obtain freer responses than can be obtained with a set pattern of questioning.

validity—refers to the ability of a data collection method or other instrument to obtain the relevant needed data or to measure what it is supposed to measure.

variable—any factor, characteristic, quality, or attribute under study.

visual analog scale (VAS)—a self-report instrument used to measure subjective experiences such as pain, nausea, fatigue and dyspnea, consisting of a line, usually 100 mm in length, with anchors at each end to indicate the extremes of the sensation under study.

χ^2—*see* chi-square.

Index